Dr. James M. Rippe's

Fit for Success

Proven Strategies for Executive Health

James M. Rippe, M.D.

Prentice Hall Press

New York   London   Toronto   Sydney   Tokyo

PRENTICE HALL PRESS
Gulf+Western Building
One Gulf+Western Plaza
New York, New York 10023

PRENTICE HALL PRESS and colophon are registered
trademarks of Simon & Schuster Inc.

Library of Congress Cataloging-in-Publication Data

Rippe, James M.
[Executive cardiofitness]
Dr. James M. Rippe's fit for success: proven strategies
for executive health / James M. Rippe.
p.   cm.
Bibliography: p.
Includes index.
ISBN 0-13-293912-6 : $19.95
1. Executives—Health programs. 2. Exercise. 3. Physical
fitness. I. Title. II. Title: Executive cardiofitness.
RA777.65.R56 1989
613—dc19   88-34140
                                                        CIP

Designed by Irving Perkins Associates, Inc.

Manufactured in the United States of America

10 9 8 7 6 5 4 3 2 1

First Edition

Acknowledgments

While it is not possible to cite all of the individuals who provided advice and support during the two-and-a-half years it took to complete this book, several deserve special recognition for their significant contributions.

Over the past 10 years, I have been fortunate to have the friendship, support, and critical judgment of a number of writers and editors. Bradford W. Ketchum, Jr., editor of *The Walking Magazine* and former senior editor of *Inc.* magazine, encouraged me to pursue this book and provided editing skills and business insights at all stages of manuscript preparation. Lillian F. Ketchum, a freelance editor, helped significantly with the book's organization. T. George Harris, editor-in-chief of *American Health* and *Psychology Today,* challenged and clarified my thinking about the mind/body interface, while Paul Aron, my editor at Prentice Hall Press, pushed me when needed, cajoled me when necessary, and never lost faith in the importance of this project.

I am also indebted to my colleague, Dr. Ann Ward, research director of the University of Massachusetts Medical Center's Exercise Physiology Laboratory, who designed the computer data base for the executive survey. Kim Bertagnoli, an exercise physiologist and research assistant, coordinated the survey mailing and led the team that tabulated and analyzed its results. Of particular help in the statistical analysis, Rob Coleman took six months off from his medical school studies to get the research underway; Dr. Robert Goldberg guided the initial epidemiological design of the project; and Stephanie O'Hanley coordinated the completion of the data base.

My professional colleagues at the UMass Department of Medicine lent consistent support. Dr. Joseph Alpert, chief of cardiology, was an early mentor at Harvard Medical School and has continued to fuel my interest in preventive cardiology. Dr. James Dalen, former chief of medicine at UMass and now Dean of the University of Arizona Medical School, spearheaded the drive to establish the UMass Center for Health and Fitness where faculty from all disciplines can explore the interface between fitness and health. Dr. Ira Ockene, professor of cardiology, provided input in a variety of medical areas, while Dr. Harry Greene, director of the Division of General Medicine, was particularly helpful on the topics of physical examinations and avoidance of cancer risks.

Numerous other colleagues served as valuable sounding boards. Dr. Patty Freedson, associate professor in the Department of Exercise Science at UMass/Amherst and a longtime research colleague, helped critique and refine ideas and content for the book. Sherri Evenson, John Porcari, Sharon Wilkie, and other staff members at my exercise physiology laboratory contributed key insights from their perspectives as exercise physiologists. Diane Morris, Ph.D., R.D., director of nutrition at the UMass Medical School Exercise Physiology Laboratory was kind enough to review the sections on nutrition.

My responsibilities and commitments as a full-time cardiologist and part-time researcher, teacher, and writer require meticulous attention to details and schedules. With much appreciation, I applaud Elizabeth Porcaro, my editorial assistant, who coordinated every phase of the research and manuscript production. Jane Hodgkinson and Mary Ann Falvey, two superb assistants, kept patient and office activities moving forward with patience and good humor, during the research and writing of this book.

Beyond such friends and colleagues, I am also indebted to the 1,139 chief executive officers, presidents, and executive vice-presidents who, by completing the eight-page questionnaire on their health and fitness practices, contributed an invaluable resource for this book. I am particularly grateful to the 40 senior executives who participated in personal interviews. The in-depth discussions provided substantive, first-person examples and anecdotes essential to understanding executives' views of health, fitness, life, and business. A list of the executives interviewed appears in appendix B (see page 193).

To all of these individuals and the many others who helped along the way, my heartfelt gratitude. The final product reflects the strength, commitment, and idealism of those who made it possible.

—James M. Rippe, M.D.
Boston, Massachusetts, 1988

Contents

Introduction   xi

1 How Are America's Executives Keeping Fit?   1

2 Exercise: The Heart of the Matter   16

3 Setting Up Your Own Exercise Program   30

4 Nutrition: Diets for a Lifetime   70

5 Managing Stress   98

6 Optimizing Your Health and Fitness   122

7 Setting Up a Corporate Program   142

8 View from the Top   156

Epilogue   177

Appendix A: Methodology: Executive Health
               and Fitness Survey   180

Appendix B: Executive Interviews   193

References   196

Index   209

Introduction

I push the timing button on my watch and take off at a slow, almost cautious pace. By the time I reach the end of the driveway, 50 yards away, my arms are part of the rhythm. I turn left and head for Commonwealth Avenue and the Boston Marathon's notorious Heartbreak Hill. Within a quarter of a mile my breathing has fit in rhythmically with my normal pace, and my mind turns to the task at hand. I begin turning sentences over in my head. I feel comfortable. It is, after all, a ritual I've followed every day for the past 20 years. The venues have varied, as have the sports, but the experience has remained the same—exercise as a type of freedom, a release valve for working things out, a road to enhanced performance and creativity.

I turn left on Commonwealth Avenue and begin to chug up the final incline on Heartbreak Hill. With thoughts of getting back to the office, I start juggling work schedules and publishing deadlines in my head. The day is hot and the hill is steep. Sweat streams down my face and begins to drip across my chest and running shorts. It may be liberating, but it's also hard work.

Somewhere, some time ago, on one of these runs I began to think about this book. I've been an athlete all my life—never a top competitor, but a regular exerciser committed to an active life-style. What has made it so appealing? As a cardiologist, I know it's good for my heart. Yet that's not the major force that drives me to jog in snow at subfreezing temperatures or tackle Heartbreak Hill on the hot, humid days of summer. Rather, it's something more immediate, almost visceral—the sense that it makes a difference from day to day. Whenever I hear a person describing his or her addiction to physical activity, the experience rings true for me—both physically and psychologically. There is no question in my mind that an active life-style is linked to one's ability to perform.

In my clinical practice as a cardiologist at the University of Massachusetts Medical Center and as director of its Exercise Physiology Laboratory, I work with many executives. Within 15 miles of our offices are corporate giants such as Data General, Digital Equipment, and Prime Computer, as well as a host of smaller bioengineering and high-technology firms. The hottest young athletic footwear companies in America, Reebok and Rockport, are also just down the road. Through the lab, we routinely provide advice to executives on how to start physical fitness programs.

About five years ago, the seeds for this book began to take root when we noticed a steadily increasing number of executives who were already physically active but who sought ways to maximize the health benefits of their exercise programs. Here was a group of fitness buffs who wanted to be even fitter. I began to ask them why they exercise, and virtually every executive described experiences similar to my own. The words were different and the exercises and life-styles were diverse, but the message was always the same. It was a message of linkage: the link between their health and fitness practices and their high level of performance. These executives not only exercised but also made changes in their diets and daily habits to maintain their health.

Were these individuals unusual? Are other executives as concerned about the link between fitness and performance? What do they do, if anything, to stay fit in the face of the unique demands created by their jobs—constant time pressures, travel, business meals, stress, the threat of "burnout" life-styles? Little research has been done on the health and fitness habits of executives, primarily because they are regarded as remote and inaccessible, too busy to be bothered with such topics. It is generally assumed that questionnaires and interview requests are intercepted at secretaries' desks. Recognizing the need for data on executive health practices, our exercise physiology lab launched the research project that forms the basis of this book.

In the fall of 1986, we mailed questionnaires to more than 3,000 top executives whose names were obtained from Dun's Marketing Services,

Fortune, Inc., and *Venture* (see appendix A, page 180). The net response of 37% was beyond all expectations. A total of 1,139 executives returned the eight-page questionnaire. The respondents included 481 top executives from Dun's list of large companies and 457 from Dun's list of small companies, 128 chief executive officers (CEOs) from the *Fortune* 500, 46 from the *Inc.* 100, and 27 from *Venture*. Most of the responses were detailed, punctuated with comments and exclamation points.

Clearly, we touched a nerve at the highest level of corporate America. We also created the first major summary of health and fitness attitudes and practices among top executives. Given the enthusiastic response, we delved into firsthand experiences through personal interviews. Thirty-three senior executives and seven health/fitness directors from 24 companies subsequently granted interviews ranging from 45 minutes to two-and-a-half hours (see appendix B, page 193). Diverse as they were in industries and interests, they had several characteristics in common. Here were deeply committed, caring people, as passionately involved with their families and friends as with their careers. In short, "people" people eager to reach out and communicate.

The survey respondents were predominantly male (97%), averaging slightly more than 50 years in age. Those representing the newer, more entrepreneurial *Inc.* and *Venture* firms were the youngsters, with an average age of 45; *Fortune* 500 executives were the seniors, at 54. Not surprisingly, the group is well educated and well compensated. More than 80% have bachelor degrees and 36% have advanced degrees, including 16% with MBAs and 10% with doctorates. Their average salaries in 1986 ranged from $141,261 among Dun's small-company executives to $356,029 for *Fortune* 500 top management. Overall, the executives' annual salaries averaged $191,539, with total annual income averaging $332,711.

Company size varied widely, from the *Inc.* contingent's average sales of $68 million to the *Fortune* group's $3 billion. Among the respondents overall, average sales were $480 million. In terms of employees, the smaller companies averaged 777 employees, while the largest—the *Fortune* 500—averaged 25,425. Overall, the average number of employees was 3,546.

Regardless of personal background or company size, however, the executives represented a powerful group of decision-makers who share much in common when it comes to attitudes about health and fitness. America's top managers, for example, are planners. They plan for their companies. But they also plan very carefully for "time out" with their families, vacations, recreation, and personal health and fitness regimes. For most, regular exercise is taken as seriously as any other appointment on their calendar. In short, the link between a high level of fitness and increased energy, stamina, and productivity is critical to them. Their concerns about their health extend into such areas as cardiovascular fitness, proper nutrition, stress reduction, and risk factor reduction.

In many ways, these executives resemble the elite athletes we have worked with in our exercise physiology laboratory—Olympic and professional athletes in sports such as rowing, marathon running, weight lifting, racewalking, and even professional baseball. While the goals for these athletes differ from those of the executives, many of the underlying characteristics are similar: discipline, consistency, attention to detail, competitiveness, and a fierce desire to excel.

Almost two-thirds of the executives in our survey exercise at least three or more times a week, compared with only 20% of the American adult population estimated by the U.S. Public Health Service to be regular exercisers (that is, the number of people who exercise enough to derive important health benefits). While this is an admirably bright picture for executives, they still have a way to go. Many are still struggling with how to get into, and stick with, a regular fitness program. Some are trying to get back to an established program. Still others are already committed to fitness but want to fine-tune their routine. An amazing 90% of the executives indicated that they would like to improve their physical condition over the next five years.

The fitness movement has spawned reams of literature on exercise prescription. Yet it is my experience with executives, confirmed by our survey and interviews, that significant knowledge gaps remain. For example, more than one-third of the executives rely on personal experience to chart their exercise programs. As a start, this isn't bad. Informed knowledge of one's own body is a worthwhile goal. Yet what struck me as I talked to many executives was that they are still functioning on information provided by the "old coach" from high school or college days. Our knowledge of exercise physiology and types of programs that can maximize health and fitness benefits has exploded during the past decade. What the old coach recommended for a young athlete is likely not the best advice for a 50-year-old executive and may actually be doing some harm to muscles and bones. Other knowledge gaps relate to dietary habits and basic facts about one's physical condition. Do you know, for example, your actual blood pressure? Your cholesterol level? You should.

In addition to the information and insights gleaned from our study, I have drawn upon extensive medical and scientific literature as source material for this book (see references, page 196). I have also drawn upon my own clinical experiences and those of my colleagues in various fields of medicine. Many of the exercise guidelines come from our own laboratory studies and more than 30 papers and books on athletic achievement, physiology, and fitness that we have published during the past three years.

Will the knowledge, experience, and advice imparted here by executives and practitioners inspire others in the corporate corridors to adopt active and healthy life-styles? I certainly hope so. But it all depends on leadership and communication. More than 50% of all medications prescribed by physicians, for example, are taken incorrectly or not at all. Clearly there's a communication problem, and it's even more severe with exercise prescriptions. Less than 20% of physicians discuss exercise with their patients. And even those who do often make it a perfunctory afterthought—"you should get more exercise."

Executive health and fitness should be a partnership between the medical profession and executives concerned about their performance. Most of the advice in this book is straightforward and disarmingly simple. I'm not talking about turning lives upside down. I'm talking about making adjustments, informed decisions about risks that you are not willing to take with your health and trade-offs you are or are not willing to make to enhance your quality of life.

In some ways, this approach flies in the face of behavioral research on the limits of cognition. After all, it is argued, knowledge alone rarely changes behavior. Most people who smoke cigarettes know they should stop, and most people who don't exercise know they should start. More than increased knowledge is necessary to alter ingrained behaviors or engraft new ones. But here I'm very optimistic. My clinical experience with executives and numerous examples provided by the executives in this book suggest that they seek knowledge and try to act on it.

In the end, advice on health and fitness relies on what one CEO who quit smoking calls "shrinking your self-interest." It relies on your commitment to make certain life-style changes. That depends on personal motivation—and that's your part of the partnership.

Dr. James M. Rippe's
Fit for Success

1

How Are America's Executives Keeping Fit?

The people who are running successful companies and working hard at it really do watch their health. You don't see many overweight people with high blood pressure running entrepreneurial companies. They take care of themselves, they're careful about what they eat, and they care about exercise.

—DONALD STEEN, president and CEO
Medical Care International, Inc.

The once widely held image of the corpulent corporate executive— rooted to a leather chair, chomping on a cigar or cigarette, enjoying three-martini lunches, and fitting in occasional midweek golf or tennis games at the country club—can now be declared a complete myth. Those at the top of the corporate ladder are the first to confirm this.

In our survey of 1,139 chief executives, we found that 64% exercise regularly, only 10% smoke (compared with the national average of almost 30%), more than 90% pay attention to their diet, 81% have had a complete physical examination within the past two years, and more than 65% know their blood pressure (which averages an excellent 124/79 mm Hg). When asked to assess their current health, a resounding 83% characterize it as very good or excellent; a nearly unanimous 98% rank their health as good, very good, or excellent. In fact, only 19 respondents consider their health just fair and only 2 report poor health.

Other results of the study support the executives' positive assessment. Consider the number of sick days, for example. On average, the executives were sick only slightly more than two days in the past year. More telling, 73% were ill two or fewer days and an incredible 52% were not sick a single day. The average amount of time lost due to illness is slightly more than one day, with 66% indicating that they had not missed a single day of work in the previous year.

The survey results and personal interviews with the respondents clearly show that America's senior executives are a remarkably healthy group that is committed to maintaining health and vigor. "Executives pay more attention to their health than any other segment of society," declared Thomas Hourihan, vice-president of human resources of the Norton Company. "They're more conscious of how important it is." Donald Steen, president and chief executive officer (CEO) of Medical Care International (MCI), agreed: "The people who are running successful companies and working hard at it really do watch their health. They take care of themselves, they're careful about what they eat, and they care about exercise. It shows that no matter how busy you are you have time to do that."

Most executives consider their health critical to functioning day to day. "If you're not in good health, you can't be successful in anything you do. Being healthy is more important than almost anything else. You can get up every day and go fight the battle. It's tough enough, but if you're sick most of the time or don't feel well, you're just not going to be up to it," observed Terry Jacobs, chairman of Jacor Communications.

Gerald Gilbert, former president and CEO of Winnebago Industries, echoed similar sentiment: "I start with a set of goals for myself—personal and financial, business and achievement goals—things I want to see and do. I don't have a specific health goal other than the knowledge that without good health my other goals are unattainable. I know it's going to require good health to get there."

That top managers put a premium on their health is no surprise. But how do they maintain it? What is most important to them in their daily lives? Asked to rank the seven chief factors that contribute to their personal health, 86% cited "not smoking" as number one. Beyond that, the top priorities are regular exercise (75%) and diet (72%). They are followed by adequate sleep (56%), controlling stress (55%), allowing time for leisure/recreation (50%), and limiting alcohol consumption (50%).

Three of four executives consider regular exercise a cornerstone to achieving and maintaining good health. "A desk-chair executive is never a successful executive," emphasized Robert Rowan, chairman and for-mer CEO of Fruehauf. "I don't care how you do it—walking through the plant or whatever—the key is to get the exercise."

"I know that if I exercise regularly it's a lot easier for me to live my life, both professionally and personally," added Charles Clough, president, chairman, and CEO of Nashua Corporation.

Richard Snyder, chairman and CEO of Simon & Schuster, attested to the importance of consistency: "There's no question in my mind," he noted. "I wouldn't be where I am today or doing the job I'm doing if it weren't for the physical aspect—my workout—that I developed in the last thirteen to fourteen years."

Most executives, in fact, make exercise an integral part of their life-styles. "I won't give it up until I have to," insisted K. W. Reese, executive vice-president at Tenneco, Inc. "I'm going to jog and run and exercise until my body tells me I can't—I'm not going to stop even if I have to get in a wheelchair to do it. Exercise is that important. The worse thing that could happen to me would be for something to happen [so] that I couldn't exercise."

Impressive in their level of commitment to exercise, these executives are also notable for the diversity of activities they pursue. Of 1,139 respondents to the survey, 64% indicated that they exercise regularly, pursuing an average of 2.6 different activities. Very few executives rely on only one type of exercise or physical activity. They vary their routines generally because of weather, travel, and availability of facilities. If the weather precludes walking or jogging, for example, they might work out on a treadmill or stationary cycle.

Depending on the weather and his business schedule, Jacor Commu-nications's Terry Jacobs spends a half hour to an hour six days a week in a program that variously consists of calisthenics, jogging, weight lifting, and working out on a cross-country ski machine. "I've experimented with lots of things," said Jacobs, "and I change the routine occasionally to avoid getting bored."

The survey's list of 17 possible activities underestimated the diverse interests of the executives, who cited more than 40 other activities they regularly pursue. Among them are gardening, hiking, horseback rid-ing, ice hockey, softball, stair climbing, and volleyball.

Avner Parnes, former chairman and CEO of MBI Business Centers, Inc., can climb 88 stairs to his office or take the elevator. "Most of the

3

time—in two out of three cases—I walk up or down the stairs, some-times three or four times a day," he explained, noting that he does it strictly for the exercise. "It gets me moving just a little bit more."

Among the executives overall, the two most popular activities are jogging/running and tennis, followed closely by golf, fitness walking, weight training, and stationary cycling. However, the list changes some-what when the activities are ranked by frequency of participation. Among those activities in which executives participate three or more times a week, the leader is jogging/running, followed by fitness walking, stationary cycling, calisthenics, and weight training. Only 19 out of 1,139 respondents play tennis three or more times a week and only four play golf that often, and both sports are surpassed by racquetball, with 22 regular players.

Particularly noteworthy is that 90% of executives who exercise three or more times a week include an activity specially designed for aerobic conditioning as a cornerstone of their fitness programs. Also significant is the number of executives (28%) who supplement their aerobic work-outs with weight-training regimens. Jogging and fitness walking are the dominant forms of aerobic exercise, with stationary cycling and calis-thenics close behind. Other common forms of aerobic exercise—swim-ming, rowing, and aerobic dance—do not have as large a following, each having about one-fifth the number of practitioners as walking or jogging. Nonetheless, aerobics excercise has a dedicated following. Al-most two out of three who participate in aerobic activities do so three or more times a week.

When describing their exercise routines, executives express a wide range of personal preferences and choice of programs, often depend-ing on individual needs and what they believe works best for them. Two other important considerations are efficiency and logistical ease. "It's important to have a sport or exercise that you can do easily," observed Charles Clough, president, chairman, and CEO of Nashua Corpora-tion. "Sure, golf is enjoyable, but it's difficult to play golf. You carry the equipment around, you block out long periods of time, and you don't get much exercise from it. Golf is not an efficient form of exercise. Tennis isn't ideal either, because you always have to find a court and partner, and if you take a trip, you end up carrying a tennis racket everywhere. If you're a businessman, you have tight schedules and you need an efficient form of exercise that you can enjoy the rest of your life, such as running or swimming."

Efficiency and convenience are the main attractions of jogging for many executives. Paul Allaire, president of Xerox Corporation, who has jogged since college ("I was into jogging before jogging began"), was quick to admit, "Running is not my favorite form of exercise, but it's an efficient one." Allaire's exercise program also includes stationary and outdoor cycling and Nautilus weight training.

"Running's so easy to do. It doesn't require equipment or facilities, and you can do it almost anywhere," said MCI's Donald Steen, who jogs three to five miles, three or four times a week. "I have an exercise machine at home that I use when I'm there, but I'm gone so often. I guess you could find clubs in different cities, but that's harder and it takes more time than just going out and running."

"I travel a lot and it's much easier to throw a pair of shoes and an outfit into the suitcase," echoed J. L. Ketelsen, Tenneco chairman and CEO, who jogs 30 minutes five days a week. "I've jogged all over the world. I've run in Beijing and just got back from Turkey. We were going to do a little sight-seeing in Ismar, and the government provided us with a guide. I happened to mention jogging, and she said, 'Oh, I'm a jogger. I'll pick you up at seven o'clock and take you jogging.' So even in a place like that, you find it's not hard to keep up with your exercising."

Two other Tenneco executives, K. W. Reese, executive vice-president, and Kenneth L. Otto, senior vice-president, are also avid joggers. Reese gets up between 5:15 and 5:30 every morning to jog three to five miles before work. Like Ketelsen and other joggers we interviewed, Reese extolled the pleasures of jogging in favorite foreign and domestic locations while on business trips. "No matter where you go, you can find a great place to run—in the hills around Zurich, along the Rhine in Germany, and even in New York City. There's no finer place than Central Park—as long as you stick to the main path."

Otto is among those who find it more challenging to set goals for themselves. "I have an objective—I'll jog one hundred miles a month. I don't care if I'm in Europe or South Africa or Japan, I run. Sometimes I can only get eighty-five in, but I'll make that up. Last year, I ran one thousand two hundred fifteen miles." Other joggers have found that setting goals detracts from the enjoyment of running. "I started off by saying I'm going to run farther. I'll run three miles, then four, then five," explained MCI's Steen. "But that started to become a pressure thing, so I decided it wasn't a good idea. I'd just run as far as I feel like running. If I can't run five miles, I won't. It works better. Trying to build up distance all the time actually provided an excuse not to do it. I'd think, 'Oh, God, I've got to run five miles. Yuck!' "

Several former joggers are now walkers. Donald Lennox, board member and former CEO of Navistar International Corp., jogged for 20 years until his heels started bothering him. "I stopped jogging and started walking as fast as I can," he said, noting that he'd get in three miles each way walking to and from work. When he can't walk, he uses a stationary cycle; he also works out with weights three or four times a week.

Avner Parnes switched to walking for a more dramatic reason. "I used to jog here (in Washington, D.C.) along the river in the mornings. There was this guy, another jogger, and we'd wave and chat with each other. Then one day I noticed he wasn't showing up anymore. I asked one of the other joggers what happened to this guy. 'You didn't hear about him?' was the reply. 'He died here; he just fell over and died.' I got scared. I just couldn't do it anymore. So I stopped jogging." Instead, Parnes started walking at least five, and sometimes seven, miles a day; and when he can't walk because of the weather, he uses a treadmill.

Many executives walk not only for the exercise but also as a way of getting outdoors with family or friends. "Very often, my wife and I exercise together," reported John Bierwirth, senior management consultant and former chairman and CEO of Grumman Corp. "I usually bicycle alone because I like to go faster than she does. But she's learned how to exercise walk. Our daughter taught her how to really step out. We don't have goals or any particular pace; we just step right out and walk. And it's a pace that most people couldn't keep up with."

To some executives, jogging, fitness walking, and other stringent exercise regimens have no appeal. "I've always said that when I see the first smiling jogger, I'll think about it. That type of exercise never appealed to me," commented Fruehauf's Robert Rowan. "I'm not the type who enjoys just working out in a gym. I like being outdoors. I love to chop wood, and I like getting away for a golf or tennis game. I need a competitive exercise or type of activity that, when finished, gives me the feeling I've accomplished something—like chopping wood, shoveling snow, raking the lawn, trimming the evergreens, weeding the flower beds, or something where I can see what I've achieved. If I can't get out and do those physical things because of my schedule, then at least I try to exercise every day."

Rowan's indoor exercise includes calisthenics and stationary cycling.

6

"I try to do just those exercises that I think help keep me physically trim—just enough every day to accelerate my heartbeat and then watch my diet to keep my weight under control," Rowan continued. "For me, that's better than a jogging program or an organized type of program."

One of the reasons swimming is not as popular among executives is the logistical factor—the availability of a pool at home, near work, on the road. Some, like Nashua's Charles Clough, have their own pool. "I commute forty-five minutes to work and find it difficult to get up in the morning and run," noted Clough. "But we have an indoor pool, and my wife and I swim every day for half an hour. I also work out on an exercise bike for another half an hour."

Another drawback with swimming, reported some executives, is boredom. Norton Company's Thomas Hourihan regards swimming as "vigorous exercise—and, one of those things that would be helpful to me that I just don't like to do. Just going back and forth in a pool drives me crazy."

Although 26 respondents to the survey indicated that they row three or more times a week, only one of the executives we interviewed, William Coors, chairman of Adolph Coors Company, relies on rowing as his main form of aerobic conditioning. "I developed a knee problem and couldn't jog anymore, so I got a rowing machine," Coors said. "Rowing is as complete an exercise as you can get. I enjoy it. Half an hour three times a week is maybe all you need, but I'm committed to exercising seven days a week."

As much as executives have individual exercise preferences, they also have varied reasons for starting and maintaining regular fitness regimens. Seventy-seven percent of the survey respondents participated in high school athletics, 46% in college, and 35% after college. Many continue to maintain a high level of physical activity, having made the transition from competitive athletics into lifetime personal programs with varying degrees of intensity, however. More than a few confess to periodic lapses in their exercise programs, particularly during their climb up the corporate ladder. "I was quite an athlete as I was growing up and I've carried those earlier health and fitness attitudes into my entire life," said Gerald Gilbert, former president and CEO of Winnebago Industries. "We all go through certain periods, though. I was extremely active up to my mid-twenties and then went through a period of being married to my job too much and using lots of excuses for not doing what I should have been doing. Then I started redeveloping that discipline," added Gilbert, who runs twice a day for 30 minutes. "If I can't run outside, I jog on a trampoline."

In a majority of cases, however, the impetus to start an exercise program or take an existing one more seriously has come from the discovery of a personal health problem, the death of a loved one or friend, or the sudden realization of being woefully out of shape. "One day I was playing on the lawn with my kids and I realized I couldn't run twenty feet without getting winded. It was the first time I realized how out of shape I had gotten. I decided right then to do what I had to do to get back in shape. Then I became addicted to exercise," explained Simon & Schuster's Richard Snyder, who started an extensive program of running, weights, and tennis that he has stuck with for more than 13 years.

Leonard Reiffel, Ph.D., CEO of Interand Corporation, had a similar awakening: "I was going to hell in a handbasket. I was getting too fat and too old, and I didn't want that to happen." As a solution, Reiffel bought a stationary cycle, which he uses four to six times a week, and started working out with weights.

"I was participating in organized sports and playing a lot of golf," said another executive, "but there came a point when I realized the games had to end and I had to find something to keep myself in reasonable shape. Between age thirty-five and forty, I started looking for more regular ways to work out. In particular, there was a two-year lull in there when I didn't have any regular physical activity. I put on some weight and my blood pressure moved up a bit. I felt a loss of energy and vitality and staying power. So I tried to find something that I would really like to do in the way of exercise. I began with the Canadian Air Force Exercise routine and then started to run. I found that I enjoyed running and started to work it into my daily schedule."

William Coors started developing what he calls a "wellness life-style" to stay in mental and physical shape when he realized he was having trouble coping with pressure. "At least thirty-five years ago, I was under a lot of pressure here. We had all kinds of problems," he explained. "I was aware that not only was I not enjoying life, but I was very, very irritated when people would bother me and very, very tired—just chronic fatigue. I'd take a short vacation and get a rest. I'd come back to the office fully refreshed and, after one hour, I was tired again. I was convinced that I was suffering from some type of obscure ailment.

Nobody realized what it was in those days, but it was nothing more than executive stress."

After undergoing a series of tests, Coors continued, "my doctor said, 'I have good news and bad news. The good news is: We can't find a damn thing wrong with you. The bad news is: There's nothing we can do for you.' He admitted that he and many of his counterparts had seen patients with the same complaints—yet, they didn't know what it was, what caused it, or how to treat it. I decided if the medical profession couldn't do much for me, I'd better see what I could do for myself."

Other executives were jolted into regular physical exercise by specific health problems. "I kept drifting away from physical activity as I got busier, spending less and less time at it. I'd gotten down to where I really didn't have any significant major sports activity," recalled Ralph Ungermann, president and CEO of Ungermann-Bass, Inc. "Then I had a very serious back problem about eight years ago and that really got me into the kick. When I came out of my operation, I decided that I was going to get myself into very good shape."

Back problems were also an incentive for Nashua's Clough: "One of the reasons that I began to exercise on a more routine basis is that I ended up with a bad back. Back problems are about the sorest things imaginable. My back starts getting sore if I don't exercise, so that's a very powerful incentive." Clough also discovered that he could "absorb a lot more stress—stay in better condition when traveling" with regular exercise. "Those are all powerful incentives," he added.

Tenneco's J. L. Ketelsen and K. W. Reese both thought they had been following acceptable exercise routines, until they encountered heart problems. Said Ketelsen, who had a coronary bypass operation in 1979, at age 52, "I wasn't uneducated about the desirability of diet and exercise before the bypass, and I thought I was keeping up with both satisfactorily. But since the bypass, my program's been more rigid and dedicated." Ketelsen switched from swimming to jogging because "it was more difficult to maintain an exercise level by swimming" and also because of travel—"it's hard to find swimming pools all the time."

Reese was very active in high school, college, and Army athletics. "Then I got into my thirties and forties. I didn't exercise as religiously as I should have, but I still continued exercising," he reported. After suffering a silent myocardial infarction in 1980, Reese got into a serious running program and started watching his diet more closely. "If I could turn back the clock ten years knowing what I know now, I know what I would have done differently. I would have changed diets and I wouldn't have driven myself so hard," reflected Reese. "Instead of working under stress, I would have learned to control stress, and the exercise program would have done that for me. If I had known enough then to exercise regularly, there's no question that the attack possibly could have been prevented."

Two other Tenneco executives, Joe B. Foster, former executive vice-president, and Kenneth L. Otto, senior vice-president, are among those whose fathers' heart attacks made lasting impressions. "I basically began exercising because my father died of heart trouble at a very early age—fifty-six. And a neighbor had an attack about the same time I turned forty," explained Foster. "I said, OK, I've really got to get serious about this, although I've been interested in athletics all my life. I simply made the commitment to exercise. It's not a philosophical thing with me—it works, and I do it."

Otto's father died of a heart attack at age 58. "He was type A, smoked Camels, had very high blood pressure, and was a reasonably successful man who chose to ignore the advice of the medical profession. He just walked in the house one night and dropped dead. That made a mark on me. I was always active physically and I've always watched my weight. As I grew up in the corporate environment, the more pressures I had, the more active I became."

Terry Jacobs had a similar experience. His father died of a heart-related ailment at an even earlier age. "My father died when he was only thirty-four," he recalled. "I was nine years old at the time, and it made a strong impression on me about trying to maintain good health. He was a very heavy smoker, probably the opposite of what I've tried to be in keeping fit." Jacobs played high school and college sports and kept exercising while working eight hours a day and attending school four hours a night. "It was tough, but I always tried to do at least ten or fifteen minutes of some type of exercise every day," he said, noting that he has sustained a program of 30 minutes to an hour a day for the past 15 years.

A number of executives in their mid- to late-fifties noted that an additional incentive to exercise is watching others who don't. In fact, one executive believes that by age 50, it's an either/or choice: "It surprises me that more people my age don't exercise. Those who do, seem to be very into it. Those who don't, don't do anything—and there's no middle ground."

"I want to keep myself in good shape because I've seen some people get sedentary in their late fifties and early sixties and I've seen others become very vigorous," said another CEO. "I have this image of where I'd like to be ten years from now—and it's doing something new and different. I want to be vigorous enough so I can call the tune for the rest of my life. That, in a nutshell, is why I exercise."

In the minds of all exercisers is the knowledge or hope that their daily or weekly regimens, whether they enjoy them or not, will help them live longer. But the motivation for exercising goes far beyond extended life span. When asked to rank the chief reasons they exercise regularly, executives rated health benefits highest. Other major motivators are improved sense of well-being, weight loss/control, improved physical appearance, reduced stress, and improved productivity. Among those factors less prominent in most executives' decisions to exercise is "enjoyment of exercise."

Consistently, the executives interviewed linked their regular exercise programs to better health, increased energy and stamina, and—a significantly unanimous theme—simply feeling good about themselves. Robert Rechholtz, vice-president of sales and markiting of Adolph Coors Company, summed it up when he described the changes he experienced: "I've always been fairly active. But until about eight years ago, I didn't pursue it on a consistent, seven-day basis. I made it a goal to work out every day, aerobically, at least for thirty minutes. After three months, I felt better, lost weight, looked better, had more energy, and felt less stress. It's the sheer ability to help yourself feel good, look good, and therefore have more confidence in your ability to compete and to associate with the rest of the world."

Said another executive: "Health and being able to look in the mirror and feel proud of myself—those are the two motivators."

It's more than greater endurance and better physical appearance that motivates these executives; it's also the ability to think more clearly and creatively. "What I find so interesting about exercise is how much sharper my mind is. I do a lot of public speaking. I often begin to think about a speech when I'm exercising and it's amazing how it helps my creative thinking," said William Coors. Echoed Donald Lennox: "If I take a forty-five- to fifty-minute walk in the morning, I come into the office with a good head of steam built up and a clear mind. I seem to be able to accomplish more. I have no tendency to sit and be drowsy. I'm ready to go."

Kenneth L. Otto's observations are also typical: "My energy level is improved. I can be at my desk by seven A.M. . . . and if I run at noon, I can hang in there until seven or eight o'clock at night. My thinking is clear, and I'm not mentally exhausted. So my exercise program has been one of the best things I've ever done."

Not all executives surveyed enjoy their routine exercise programs: About two out of five confess that they occasionally have problems sticking with them. When asked to indicate the primary factors that hinder or limit them from maintaining regular exercise, they cited travel and disruptive schedules most often, followed by inadequate time and lack of motivation.

Many executives described the difficulties encountered in maintaining their exercise programs while traveling—the demands of airline schedules, early and late meetings, social obligations, jet lag—and how they overcome these problems. "Travel doesn't inhibit my exercise because I don't let it. I ask to be put in a hotel that has a pool or a place nearby where I can run," explained Charles Clough. "It's not that difficult to arrange, and a little preplanning can make an enormous difference."

Some executives use exercise to overcome travel weariness. "When I'm traveling and I'm tired, I absolutely force myself to exercise," explained Ralph Ungermann. "It helps me endure the tiredness and strain. Even if I get to bed late, I wake up early and go for at least a short run. It just makes me feel better when I do that."

Other frequent travelers, like Donald Steen, have adopted specific strategies to minimize the disruptions of travel: "It's easier if you stick with places you know. If you stay in the same hotels in New York or San Francisco, you can get up and run because you know where you are. . . . I try to control both where I stay and what my schedule demands. If I know I'm going to have a late dinner meeting, then I don't schedule a breakfast meeting for the next morning. I allow myself some time so I can get up and exercise."

Even if not traveling, the daily interruptions of meetings and other commitments are impediments to regular exercise. While solutions to this problem vary, they are often quite simple, requiring a little planning and discipline. Many executives have simply established a regular time when they exercise. Some, like Tenneco's Ketelsen and Reese and Jacor's Jacobs, prefer the morning. "I found that if I didn't get up and exercise early in the morning before going to the office, too many other things got in the way," explained Jacobs. Others, like Ronald Thomas, chairman and former president of Ciprico, Inc., prefers noontime, "because I'm not an early riser and later in the evening it gets too dark to run."

Richard Snyder of Simon & Schuster has found that scheduling his exercise sessions as if they were regular business appointments minimizes the likelihood of external interruptions. "My secretary is trained to move my schedule around to make sure I can get my workout in," said Snyder. "Whatever it takes, that time is mine. . . . You have to justify that you can do that, that it's also good for the company. The healthier and stronger I am, the more relaxed I am, the better it is for the company."

Among those who exercise regularly, one of the incentives for keeping up their exercise schedules is what happens when they become less active. "If I don't get any exercise for a period of time, and particularly if I eat too much during that period, I put on a couple of pounds and just plain slow down," lamented John Bierwirth. "It's just not good."

Several executives noted that, as they get older, if they go for even just a few days without exercising, it is harder to get back in shape. "When I exercise regularly, I find a distinct difference. Not just a subtle difference, a distinct difference. I feel fit and other things happen, like improvements in my energy level and staying power. I sleep better. I eat less. I feel like I'm twenty-five again," said Norton's Thomas Hourihan. "When I go the other route and somehow get off my exercise pattern, I notice it's harder to concentrate for long periods of time. I don't sleep as well and I certainly don't have the stamina or energy. There's a real drop. Now that I'm going on fifty-three, I suspect there's more of a drop-off than there was ten or fifteen years ago."

A few of the executives we interviewed were in sustained "drop-off" periods. They were not exercising regularly and hadn't for some time, even though they were keenly aware of the benefits. How, we asked the regular exercisers and nonexercisers alike, can top managers be so effective at controlling their business lives and yet fail to control other aspects of their lives? "I don't know what it is; I've used all kinds of rationalizations," admitted one nonexerciser. "In the summertime, I play golf a lot, but then there are those months . . . I won't do anything and yet I know I'd feel better by exercising."

The most common theme tied to the failure to exercise, however, was the press of business, particularly among younger executives trying to make their mark or run their own companies. "Succeeding in business has taken a toll on my ability to maintain my health and fitness," said one executive. "When I worked for someone else, I exercised daily. I'd run three miles a day. . . . I would ski at least fifteen to twenty-five days a year. Now that I manage a company with fifty people, I don't have time for that. I didn't use to have to worry about the bills getting out or whether ten people in the office were feuding with each other. Now the entire universe is my responsibility—and that's my exercise."

While acknowledging similar business pressures in their careers, the regular exercisers don't accept such excuses. "It's very simple," said one executive. "You can always do what you decide to do. All you have to do

EXECUTIVE HEALTH: ATTITUDES AND MOTIVATORS
(PERCENT OF RESPONDENTS TO EXECUTIVE SURVEY)

	Not important	Average importance	Very important
HEALTH ATTITUDES			
Not smoking	5%	8%	87%
Regular exercise	5	19	76
Diet (less sugar, salt, fat)	6	21	73
Adequate sleep	11	33	56
Controlling stress	10	35	55
Limiting alcohol consumption	10	39	51
Allowing for leisure/recreation	15	34	51
MOTIVATING FACTORS			
Health benefits	3	10	87
Improved sense of well-being	6	20	74
Maintain/lose weight	10	19	71
Improved physical appearance	8	28	64
Reduced stress	18	26	56
Improved productivity	16	31	53
Enjoyment of exercise	25	24	51
Better equipped to tackle problems	26	30	44
Increased concentration	33	30	37
Improved appetite	65	19	16

Source: Compiled by the author.

14

is decide." Commented another CEO when told by some employees that they didn't have time to exercise: "Nonsense. You make your own priorities."

When asked why he thinks executives who know they should be exercising don't exercise, Tenneco's Ketelsen replied: "Business executives are no different than anybody else. They're guys who know they ought to be doing something but they just aren't going to do it, they just don't have the time to worry about that part of it. But, it's changing . . . the trend toward fitness is very strong. You're going to see more and more emphasis on it, and it's going to be harder and harder to duck it.

"It just takes an hour extra," Ketelsen added. "I get up an hour earlier than I'd like to get my exercise in. There isn't any other answer to it."

EXECUTIVE EXERCISE/PHYSICAL ACTIVITY PREFERENCES

Activity	Percent who participate	Percent who participate three or more times per week
Jogging/running	35%	72%
Tennis	35	7
Golf	32	2
Fitness walking	31	66
Stationary cycling	27	64
Weight training	27	56
Calisthenics	18	94
Racquetball	12	26
Outdoor cycling	10	10
Aerobic dance/exercise	8	36
Downhill skiing	7	N/A
Swimming	6	88
Rowing	5	67
Cross-country skiing	5	11
Basketball	3	24
Squash/handball	2	19
Bowling	2	0
Other	10	30

Source: Compiled by the author.

2

Exercise: The Heart of the Matter

You can't do a good job if you don't have the strength and stamina to cope with the many problems you face every day. Your mind won't work better than your body in the long run.

—ROBERT ROWAN, chairman and
former CEO
Fruehauf

Scientific and medical research long ago documented the linkages between daily habits and lifetime health, and the evidence is irrefutable: People who exercise live longer.

This conclusion is further supported by the ongoing College Alumni Study begun in 1962 and led by epidemiologist Dr. Ralph S. Paffenbarger, Jr., of the University of California at San Francisco. The study shows that individuals who walk an average of five city blocks a day, climb five flights of stairs daily, or engage in 30 minutes of vigorous sports play a day are significantly less likely to suffer a heart attack or sudden death than their more sedentary counterparts. Even more important, by the time these individuals reach their seventies, they live an average of two years longer than nonexercisers.

A wealth of anecdotal experience demonstrates that exercisers enjoy a higher *quality* of life; the College Alumni Study adds proof that physical activity also extends the *quantity* of life. Equally strong evidence underscores the negative impact of poor health practices. Cigarette smokers, for example, are 30 times more likely than nonsmokers to develop lung cancer and three times as likely to incur heart disease. Elevated cholesterol and blood pressure independently expose the individual to twice the risk of heart disease. Even more alarming is evidence

16

that risk factors multiply—rather than simply add to—each other. An individual with high cholesterol and elevated blood pressure who smokes is 8 times more likely to develop heart disease than an individual with none of these risk factors.

While the impact of personal habits on health is self-evident, the relationship between exercise and job performance is not so obvious. Executives often ask what happens to their bodies when they exercise. Physical activity triggers a number of physiologic processes, some immediately, some within a minute or so, and still others within 5 to 10 minutes. This is because the body has two major systems for generating the energy required for exercise and all other daily activity. The systems are called "aerobic" and "anaerobic."

Aerobic literally means "in the presence of air." This system combines carbon-containing fuels in the body, such as glucose, with oxygen carried in the bloodstream to generate the molecules needed to supply energy. The aerobic energy system is the body's primary energy producer. It is responsible for virtually all of the energy that maintains the body at rest and more than 90% of the energy produced during exercise—except during short bursts of intense exertion.

The anaerobic system generates energy in the absence of oxygen. Even at rest, a small portion of energy comes from this source. Its major roles, however, occur during the first minute of exercise, before an increased amount of oxygen-rich blood can reach the exercising muscles, and during short bursts of high-intensity exercise when the demand for energy briefly overwhelms the capacity of the aerobic system.

If you consider the body analogous to an automobile, the aerobic system is like the regular carburization system for the engine. The anaerobic system serves as a kind of fail-safe system or booster pump to allow short bursts of intense energy. The aerobic output is by far the most efficient. When the anaerobic system kicks in, it allows increased energy production, but it also generates a lot of waste products because it is so much less efficient.

What happens, then, when you begin exercising? Let's say you are about to spend 20 minutes jogging, fitness walking, or working out on a stationary cycle. As you take your first step or perform the first pedal revolution, the exercising muscles immediately begin to expend energy to contract and call on the heart and lungs to deliver more oxygen-rich blood. It takes 45 to 90 seconds for the increased quantities of oxygenated blood pumped out by the heart to reach the exercising muscles.

During this time, your muscles rely on local energy supplies while your body slowly shifts from anaerobic to aerobic energy production.

By the time you reach the two- to three-minute mark (about a quarter-mile for most joggers), energy production stabilizes with more than 90% coming from the aerobic processes. As long as you maintain a steady pace and exercise within your appropriate capacity, energy production will be very stable and your workout will remain comfortable.

At the end of your exercise, as you taper off, energy production declines slowly; however, energy consumption remains somewhat elevated for several minutes after you stop. This time period is sometimes called "oxygen debt" to suggest that you are "paying back" some of the initial anaerobic metabolism used at the beginning of your exercise and, to a much smaller degree, throughout your workout.

Besides providing insights into your energy levels, understanding the physiology of exercise will also help you appreciate the importance of gradual warm-up and cool-down periods. During the first few minutes of exercise, your heart and lungs are struggling to catch up with the needs of the exercising muscles. Sudden strenuous exercise, without proper warm-up, will, at the least, be very uncomfortable, since you force your body to become deeply anaerobic and generate large amounts of waste. Sudden strenuous exercise can even be dangerous, since you force your heart to jump from its normal resting state to intense activity without proper warm-up.

Cooling down is no less important. During peak exercise, subtle changes occur in the blood vessels. For example, many of the vessels to the muscles dilate to facilitate blood flow to areas where it is needed most. After the workout, your heart and cardiovascular system are easing back into the resting state. A gradual cool-down allows vessels to constrict, blood flow to be redirected, and normal, slower rhythm to resume. At the same time, proper cool-down also helps your body rid itself of wastes that have accumulated during exercise.

Whether for competitive athletes or competitive executives, certain types of activities and sports are classified as "aerobic," since they are ideal for conditioning and improving the aerobic energy production system. The most common aerobic exercises, and the ones I recommend, are fitness walking, jogging or running, swimming, and cycling (outdoor or stationary). Rowing (outdoors or on an indoor machine), cross-country skiing (outdoors or on a simulator), and aerobic dance are also excellent aerobic exercises. The underlying similarity among all of these forms of exercise is the use of large muscle groups in repetitive fashion.

When an inactive executive initiates an aerobic exercise program, or increases an existing one, important physiological changes occur. These changes, which reliably occur during an 8- to 12-week period, include an increase in work capacity, less fatigue at any level of work, and a decrease in resting heart rate. Together, these changes are called the "training effect." Hundreds of scientific studies have demonstrated that these changes occur in men and women of any age, providing they follow an appropriately high level of exercise on a regular basis for 8 to 12 weeks.

There are four criteria for achieving a training effect. The exercise must be:

1. Aerobic
2. Consistent (I generally recommend 3 to 5 times per week)
3. Intense (enough to elevate the heart rate to 60% to 85% of predicted maximum)
4. Continuous (20 to 60 minutes per session)

These four guidelines have been adopted by the American Heart Association and the American College of Sports Medicine as a prescription for aerobic exercise. Some exercise physiologists summarize the last three guidelines as FIT: Frequency 3 to 5 times per week), Intensity (60% to 85% of maximum heart rate), and Time (20 to 60 minutes).

As you develop a consistent pattern of aerobic exercise, you begin to establish regular times when you call on your heart and exercising muscles to work harder. Over an 8- to 12-week period, both become more efficient. The heart becomes more productive in terms of pumping larger volumes of oxygenated blood (in medical parlance, the "cardiac output" increases).

One manifestation of this increased efficiency is the decrease in resting heart rate that individuals experience shortly after starting an exercise program. Since the more efficient heart pumps out more oxygenated blood per beat, fewer beats are required per minute. As Dr. Paul Dudley White, the father of American cardiology, said, "Every human heart is programmed at birth for a certain number of beats."

19

Most cardiologists agree that it is healthier to take those beats with a trained heart at 55 beats per minute than at an untrained rate of 80 beats per minute.

Another physiological change that occurs with training is the increased efficiency with which exercising muscles extract oxygen from the blood. Thus, while the heart muscle is growing stronger, the exercising muscles are growing more efficient, reducing the load on the heart since more oxygen can be extracted per unit of blood pumped out. While this adaptation to exercise is important to anyone who wants to improve cardiovascular endurance, it is critical to patients with coronary heart disease who have angina or have suffered a heart attack. The load that is taken off the heart by the increased efficiency of exercised muscles is often the key to resuming an active life.

While exercise physiology may seem a bit arcane, it underlies the improved energy levels and sense of well-being you experience once you launch an aerobic exercise program and stick with it.

"I made it a goal to work out every day aerobically for thirty minutes," reported Robert Rechholtz, vice-president of sales and marketing of Adolph Coors Company. "After about three months, the benefits become obvious. I lost weight, I felt better, looked better, had more energy and less stress. So I continued the workouts, and after about six months it got even better. I plateaued at about one year, but I was quite satisfied with that plateau and have remained there ever since."

The predictable training effects, which represent increased cardiovascular endurance reliably begin to occur within 8 to 12 weeks of starting an aerobic exercise program and are highly adaptive for hard-charging executives. The greater endurance, increased feelings of well-being, and control over one's body, as well as the reduced sense of stress, all contribute directly to the needs that top executives typically express.

"You may not necessarily think better, but having more stamina and being more alert is certainly a good place to start," noted Ralph Ungermann, head of Ungermann-Bass.

If lower stress, greater stamina, and an enhanced sense of well-being were the only benefits of improved cardiovascular fitness, they would easily justify prescribing aerobic exercise for every executive in America. However, there's an even greater justification or incentive, and that's the role that consistent aerobic exercise plays in reducing coronary heart disease. The link between aerobic exercise and cardiovascular health is far more than a matter of productivity; it is an issue of life and death.

By any criteria, the Western world is struggling with an epidemic of heart disease. More than 1 million individuals suffer heart attacks in the United States each year, half of whom die before they reach a hospital. In fact, more Americans die of heart disease than all other diseases combined. The problem is particularly severe in men between ages 40 and 60. In this group, heart attacks and other manifestations of narrowing of the arteries kill twice as many individuals as any other single disease. By the time a man reaches age 55, he has a 33% chance of developing symptomatic coronary artery disease. By age 60, he has a 20% chance of already having suffered a heart attack.

As a life-threatening problem facing America's executives, diseases of the heart and blood vessels can be divided into three basic categories: coronary heart disease, hypertension, and stroke.

HEART DISEASE AND ARTERIOSCLEROSIS

By far the dominant disorder is coronary heart disease (CHD), which is responsible for 87% of all annual cardiac mortality and causes almost as many deaths each year as all forms of cancer combined. The major manifestations of CHD are angina and heart attack. More than 5 million Americans currently alive have had a heart attack, angina, or both. The peak incidence for CHD occurs between ages 45 and 75, with men significantly more likely than women to suffer from it. At least 45% of heart attacks in men occur under age 65.

Most executives I see in my cardiology practice come to me because they are concerned about CHD. Either they know someone who has angina or has recently suffered a heart attack, or they're having symptoms that worry them—such as chest discomfort, excessive fatigue, or shortness of breath. I always take these concerns seriously. In some instances it is simply a matter of reassurance. In others some simple tests are required. In a few, we actually go so far as to perform heart catheterization (if the symptoms are worrisome and the screening tests are abnormal).

Some executives come to see me because they know their risk factors are high and want to do something about it. I particularly like working on this problem because often simple life-style changes can significantly reduce the risk of heart disease before signs or symptoms develop.

The underlying cause of CHD is arteriosclerosis, or thickening and hardening of the arteries that supply the heart. While considerable

21

advances have been made in identifying arteriosclerosis, medical science is still trying to pinpoint all the factors that damage the wall or inner lining of an artery. These injured areas prove to be places where arteriosclerotic plaque builds up, progressively narrowing the artery. As this process advances in any or all of the three major arteries to the heart, symptoms usually result. If the symptom reflects inadequate blood flow to the heart muscle, chest pains—angina—typically occur. If an artery becomes totally blocked off, the result is a heart attack and permanent damage to the heart muscle.

Numerous studies, including the Framingham Heart Study where more than 5,000 residents of the town of Framingham, Massachusetts, have been followed for the past 25 years, have confirmed some of the risk factors that predispose individuals to development of CHD. These have traditionally been classified as major and minor risk factors to indicate their role in the etiology of CHD.

RISK FACTORS FOR CORONARY HEART DISEASE

Major Risk Factors	Minor Risk Factors
Cigarette smoking	Inactive life-style
Elevated blood cholesterol	Family history of coronary
High blood pressure	heart disease
	Diabetes
	Stress
	Obesity

A recent analysis of previous exercise studies by the Centers for Disease Control suggests that the significance of inactivity as a cardiac risk factor has been underestimated and that it should be reclassified as a major risk of CHD. Several observations about these cardiac risk factors should be emphasized.

First, all of the major risk factors and three of the minor ones are directly under your control. Abstinence from cigarettes, regular blood pressure checks, and periodic assessment of blood cholesterol are prudent steps that should be taken by every executive. With 25% of deaths attributed to increased weight, obesity is also clearly linked to CHD. The most logical explanation relating excess weight to CHD comes from its well-documented associations with inactivity, elevated cholesterol, and high blood pressure. Counteracting the multiple hazards of inactivity, stress, and obesity requires planning, but for most top managers these programs are already in place—or could be with little change in routine.

Second, and unfortunately, keep in mind that these risk factors tend to multiply each other rather than add to each other in terms of overall CHD risk. Thus, the individual with one major risk factor has twice the risk of developing CHD compared with the individual with no risk factors. Your chances of developing CHD quadruple with two major risk factors; and if all three major risk factors are present, your risk goes up eight times. Clearly, it's best to have no risk factors, but if you have at least one (as more than 50% of executives in our survey do) it lends urgency to controlling it and minimizing the others.

Finally, risk factors tend to overlap as well. The executives in our survey who smoke cigarettes, for example, are much less likely to exercise than those who don't smoke. An inactive life-style is often associated with obesity, and obesity, in turn, is associated with both diabetes and high blood pressure. In short, the bad news about cardiac risk factors is that the slippery slope can be steep. The good news, however, is that action to reduce one risk factor can have important ripple effects on other risk factors.

HYPERTENSION

Hypertension, or high blood pressure, is one of the major risk factors for all forms of vascular disease, including CHD and stroke. Individuals with poorly controlled hypertension suffer seven times as many strokes as people with normal blood pressure (indeed, there is a history of hypertension in more than 90% of stroke victims) and more than twice as many heart attacks.

Hypertension is also the most common risk factor for vascular disease. More than 54 million Americans have high blood pressure—more than one-fifth of the population of the United States. It is a common problem among the top executives we surveyed, with at least one out of five aware that they suffer from this condition. However, the prevalence of hypertension among executives may be significantly underestimated, since an amazing 32% do not know their blood pressure.

Hypertension is one of the most easily recognizable and controllable risk factors for heart disease. It is defined as either a systolic pressure of greater than 140 millimeters (mm) of mercury (Hg) or diastolic blood pressure (BP) of greater than 90 mm Hg, or both. A more useful definition breaks down the diastolic portion of hypertension into three classifications: mild (diastolic BP 90–104 mm Hg), moderate (diastolic BP 105–114 mm Hg), and severe (diastolic BP 115 mm Hg or higher).

The exact underlying cause of hypertension has been frustratingly difficult to pinpoint, although medical science is beginning to gain clearer insights. In more than 90% of the individuals who have this disorder, no specific underlying cause can be determined. The bulk of modern research supports the concept that the problem for most individuals with hypertension is a disorder in how the kidneys handle sodium—a difficult problem since the average adult consumes twice the amount of sodium needed daily.

Two other conditions that are common in both the executive and general populations may be interrelated to hypertension. The first is obesity and the second is stress. There is no question that weight gain is related to increases in blood pressure. One of the common recommendations I give individuals with mild or even moderate hypertension is to lose weight. Often this is enough to resolve the problem without resorting to drug therapy. The relationship between stress and hypertension is more controversial, although a recent study of air traffic controllers showed that they had four times the incidence of hypertension found in the normal population.

For most executives with mild or moderate hypertension, the best way to reduce this risk factor is to pay close attention to daily life-style and habits. Salt reduction is invariably the first step. Remove the saltshaker from the table and pay close attention to reducing salt in the regular diet. This typically involves substitution of processed foods with more natural foods, such as grains, fruits, and vegetables. Weight reduction is also a mainstay of treatment, with reliance on regular exercise as a component of weight control. There may also be a place with such techniques as meditation or the relaxation response, although these are less accepted by most busy executives than salt reduction and weight control.

What's the bottom line for executives who want to effectively reduce the risk of high blood pressure? The first defense is knowledge. Have your blood pressure taken at least once a year—preferably every six months. If your blood pressure is elevated, even to a mild degree, consult your physician and follow the simple recommendations above as a painless and effective way of keeping this risk factor under control.

STROKE

Stroke is one of the leading causes of death each year in the United States, surpassed only by CHD and cancer. More than 2 million individuals currently alive have suffered strokes, making the incidence about 1%. In our survey of executives, the incidence was identical; 11 out of 1,139 respondents listed stroke as a diagnosis. Fortunately, the number of strokes has declined dramatically, dropping an average of 5% per year for the past 16 years.

The risk factors for stroke are similar to those for other forms of vascular disease. Stroke and hypertension, however, are strongly associated; more than 90% of stroke victims show a history of high blood pressure. Certain other heart conditions, such as some types of rhythm problems and certain abnormalities of the heart valves, are also associated with higher risk of stroke.

Some risk factors for stroke are beyond your control, including advancing age, being male, being black, and diabetes. A number of risks clearly can be controlled and reduced, however, including hypertension, elevated blood cholesterol, smoking, excessive alcohol intake, physical inactivity, and obesity.

In about 10% of cases, major strokes are preceded by warning symptoms that essentially result from smaller strokes. These symptoms, called transient ischemic attacks or TIAs, include:

- Unexplained dizziness, unsteadiness, or sudden falls
- Temporary loss of vision or dimness, especially in one eye
- Temporary loss of speech or difficulty understanding speech or talking
- Sudden temporary weakness of a portion of the face or one arm or leg

Each of these warning symptoms is cause for great concern and should prompt immediate medical attention.

THE EXERCISE LINK

The long-term relationship between exercise and the reduction of heart disease, hypertension, and stroke cannot be overstated. Numerous studies over the past 30 years show that individuals who are active on the job have fewer heart attacks than those who are sedentary. Early investigations were duplicated on railway workers, postal workers, and farmers with surprisingly similar results—the active workers were significantly less likely than sedentary ones to develop heart disease.

Other studies supported by the National Institutes of Health and the American Heart Association in the 1960s and 1970s continued to support the protective value of exercise. Finally, in the early 1980s, Dr. Ralph Paffenbarger and his colleagues began to release findings of their 25-year study of Harvard and University of Pennsylvania graduates. Called the College Alumni Study, it was based on long-term follow-up of more than 16,000 men.

The study clearly linked regular physical activity to reduction in heart attacks and sudden death. By the time participants reached their seventies, the regular exercisers lived an average of two years longer than their more sedentary colleagues. Of great interest is the fact that the amount of exercise required to confer substantial benefit is not large—walking an average of nine miles per week conferred substantial reductions in cardiac risk.

The College Alumni Study provided a critical piece of the puzzle relating exercise to cardiovascular fitness. It is solid evidence that life-long, consistent aerobic exercise provides important cardiac health benefits as well as enhancing day-to-day endurance and performance.

A major reason why most executives exercise is to improve their health, specifically their cardiovascular health. In our survey, 64% classified themselves as regular exercisers. Unfortunately, however, many of them have only vague impressions of how to structure their exercise programs to derive the most significant cardiac benefits. Clearly, executives are paying more attention to their daily habits in terms of exercise, nutrition, and life-style. But, the trend has also created problems and misconceptions.

Perhaps the most significant area of confusion is between the short-term cardiac *training* benefits of exercise and the long-term cardiovascular *health* benefits of an active life-style. "Training effects" are a very specific cluster of changes that occur in both the cardiovascular system and muscles. These changes include the ability to perform higher work loads and exercise for longer periods of time. The individual may also experience improved energy levels and a decrease in resting heart rate. Achieving these "training effects" requires exercising in a particular way, at a given level of intensity, for specified periods of time.

Such training benefits are very important; after all, it pays to improve endurance and energy level. However, the way one exercises to achieve training benefits may be quite different from the way one exercises to achieve long-term cardiovascular health benefits. As a cardiologist, when I think about the latter, I think primarily about the reduction in coronary heart disease.

Medical science has uncovered critical new information about how daily habits and life-style impact on the likelihood of heart disease. Some of these facts have clearly reached the highest levels of corporate America. How else can you explain, for example, the dramatic decline in cigarette smoking from 60% to the current 10% among executives in our survey?

As shown by our survey, the majority of executives exercise regularly. The problem is not lack of *general* knowledge that exercise is beneficial; it's lack of *specific* knowledge of how to structure an exercise program to optimize the cardiovascular benefits and avoid the pitfalls and potential dangers of inactivity.

In my practice of cardiology, I see a large number of executives seeking exercise programs. Sometimes they are referred by their physicians, but more often than not they refer themselves. While the specific issues are often different, the common underlying themes are similar— the desire to improve cardiovascular fitness either by initiating a new exercise program or by fine-tuning an old one. For example, the president of one of the largest travel agencies in the Northeast expressed the desire to start an exercise program. Two months before, he had lost his executive vice-president to a massive heart attack. At age 55, he was 15 pounds overweight and, except for weekend tennis, almost completely sedentary. My prescription: a walking program and diet.

In another case, a prominent attorney sought advice following a heart attack at age 43. A heart catheterization had shown narrowing of two of the arteries supplying blood to his heart. He was determined to minimize the risk of a second heart attack and rely on coronary bypass surgery only as a last resort. We devised a combined program of stationary cycling, swimming, and fitness walking, with strict attention to target heart rate. This allowed him to exercise daily with maximum benefit and minimum risk and boredom.

The president of a manufacturing firm referred himself because a painful knee had curtailed his running. The knee injury was a recurring problem resulting from a football injury 20 years before. It was fine to walk around on it, but running aggravated the chronic underlying injury. A pair of specially designed orthotics and several months of supervised physical therapy allowed him to resume running without pain.

Unfortunately, not all cases have happy endings. Some executives seek help in improving their cardiovascular health and fitness, yet never manage to adopt a consistent program. Change is hard, particularly when it involves fundamental, daily habits. Many of the executives interviewed described how difficult it had been to establish an exercise routine and how they overcame the obstacle. Often, the strategy is disarmingly simple.

"I found that if I didn't get up and exercise every morning, too many other things got in the way," reported Terry Jacobs, chairman of Jacor Communications. "So I simply established a regular time slot to get the workout in before I go to the office."

Very infrequently a serious medical problem exists that should be remedied before an exercise program can be safely pursued. Most often, these are orthopedic problems, but occasionally a serious cardiac condition requires attention before exercise can safely be prescribed. The example of a local architect is etched in my mind. He was a 51-year-old man who had suffered a heart attack at age 49. The experience had changed his life forever. He quit smoking, dropped 25 pounds, and started a regular exercise program—first through a supervised cardiac rehabilitation program at the local hospital and subsequently on his own. He eventually became a 4- to 5-mile-a-day jogger.

Things went well for a couple of years, but then he began to have a few symptoms—at first just a little more shortness of breath than he was used to and an occasional episode of mild chest pressure. Finally, one summer day, he felt dizzy during a run, had to sit down, and finally walked home. When he reported these symptoms to his physician, they were cause for great concern. A 24-hour electrocardiogram showed periods of dangerous heart rhythm disturbances, and he was referred to me.

I recommended that he stop exercising temporarily and enter the hospital so we could study the rhythm problem and start medical therapy to control it. He refused. "I've had enough of doctors and hospitals to last me a lifetime," he insisted. "The gains I've made in the last two years, I've made on my own with a good diet and exercise program. I've gotten this far on my own, and I'm not about to stop now."

A month later, he was found dead on the side of a road, dressed in his running outfit.

Fortunately, in the absence of known heart disease the incidence of sudden death during exercise is very low. In fact, it has been estimated that the average person exposes himself to more risk of death with the decision to keep driving an automobile for another year than he does with the decision to exercise for another year. Nonetheless, the architect's story underscores the simple but important message not to leave your common sense behind when you don your exercise outfit.

3

Setting Up Your Own Exercise Program

Top executives don't completely believe anyone. The real top people, the CEOs, have come to trust their own sensitivities and they retain a little distrust for everyone—even their physicians. They shop around and often try to make decisions on their own.

> —Dr. Edward J. Bernacki, vice-president, health, environmental medicine, and safety Tenneco, Inc.

One of the questions executives frequently ask is how to start an exercise program, or how to fine-tune an existing one. Even those who have well-established exercise routines are often operating with obsolete or incomplete information. Ironically, although they demand high levels of accurate information to run their businesses, executives generally do not have the same level of information on personal health and fitness.

When asked about their main sources of information on the topic, more executives cited health and sports magazines and the media (44%) than personal physicians (42%). Beyond those, previous personal experience (35%) was the only other common reference. It is not surprising that busy executives rely heavily on the media for fitness information. They are inexpensive, readily available, up-to-date, and convenient sources of information. And the advice offered can be accepted or not as the executive sees fit. Only a small minority of top managers subscribe to health newsletters or magazines. As one CEO explained the prevailing attitude, "The standard periodicals are sufficient; they're generally loaded with information on health and fitness. We're bombarded constantly with information."

What is surprising is the relatively limited reliance on personal physicians for fitness information. General distrust is one factor, points out Dr. Edward Bernacki, former medical director at United Technologies and now at Tenneco. Also, physicians have only recently started to recognize the importance of including exercise prescriptions and advice as part of routine health care. Perhaps only one out of five has detailed discussions about exercise with his or her patients and substantially fewer—certainly no more than 5%—actually spell out specific programs. Why is the role of the medical profession in this area so limited?

First, physicians receive very little instruction in medical school, or at any stage in their training, on the role of exercise in health maintenance and how to prescribe it. Most medical education is devoted to recognizing and treating disease, rather than learning how to prevent it. As a medical student in the mid-1970s, I got one lecture on exercise in four years. At most medical schools, there are no lectures for medical students on either exercise or nutrition.

Another reason physicians seldom provide a detailed exercise prescription is the time required—both for the prescription and follow-up. Few busy office practices are geared to spending the initial 45 minutes to an hour required to explain an exercise program and the periodic 30-minute consultations required to assess the patient's progress.

A third problem is finding the words and programs to help people make fundamental changes in their daily behavior. Even with a major interest in exercise, I often have difficulty finding the right combination of advice and prescribed exercise to help executives adopt positive health and fitness programs that are suitable for them and that they will stick to.

Finally, the amount physicians themselves exercise is a hurdle, although there's room for optimism. In a lecture to several hundred doctors not long ago, I asked how many exercise regularly. Only a few raised their hands, but this is changing. In a recent survey of first-year medical students at the University of Massachusetts Medical School, more than 70% indicated that they exercise regularly. The acid test will come during their internships and residencies, and during the first few years of their practices. During this period, which may span 7 to 10 years, many physicians lose control of their time and simultaneously lose touch with their bodies. The real tragedy is that doctors who don't pay attention to their own health and fitness are very unlikely to emphasize it to their patients.

One-third of the executives we interviewed started or refocused their exercise programs on the advice of physicians—prompted, however, by a rehabilitative health need, rather than as a preventative measure. Several who had been diagnosed with heart problems or who had undergone heart surgery were in cardiac rehabilitation programs prescribed by their cardiologists. One executive who had a hip replacement operation started stationary cycling as part of his therapy and subsequently consulted a cardiologist to devise a long-term program. Another executive with a back (disc) problem went to a specialty clinic and three orthopedists before settling on an exercise regimen suitable to his needs and interests.

Several executives started exercise programs of their own after reading fitness books: The Canadian Air Force Exercises and author Kenneth Cooper were the sources cited most often.

The Canadian Air Force Exercises are a series of calisthenics that can be done at home to improve both cardiovascular conditioning and muscle tone and strength. Included are such exercises as running in place, jumping jacks, sit-ups, and push-ups. These exercises were quite popular in the late 1950s and early 1960s. Much to my amazement some executives who started doing this routine in the 1960s are still keeping it up. The chief advantage of these exercises is that they require virtually no equipment and can be done in a confined space. The chief disadvantage is that they don't take full advantage of the numerous advances in knowledge and equipment that have occurred in the past 20 years.

Dr. Kenneth Cooper is a physician who practices in Dallas. His first book *Aerobics,* published in the mid-1960s, took information well known to exercise physiologists and showed the important links between exercise and health. Cooper also made an important contribution by reducing exercise regimens to a practical "point" system to help people quantify their programs.

Some executives, like Simon & Schuster's Richard Snyder, sought outside advice before launching their programs. "I didn't know the first thing to do, so I consulted an exercise physiologist who gave me a program and built me up slowly as I developed my stamina," explained Snyder. "That's the program I still follow, although I stopped with the physiologist long ago—once I got the program I was satisfied with and saw a change. You learn to go with how your body feels."

Even when outside counsel is provided, some executives prefer to do their own thing, as Robert Rowan discovered when he set up an executive health center in Fruehauf's office complex. "Initially, I had a health programmer come in to set up an exercise program for anyone who was interested," he noted. "But I soon found that most people preferred to establish their own programs, so we discontinued the health center."

In talking with executives about their fitness routines, I am always struck by the number who base their exercise routines solely on personal experience and advice that goes back to school and college days.

Now, I don't oppose tradition, but it often gets in the way of progress and in the area of exercise can even be dangerous. For example, take the old coach's saw about not drinking water while you exercise. Poor advice at best and also dangerous. It led a whole generation of athletes to suffer needless discomfort during workouts. Modern research clearly shows withholding water causes declines in performance. In some instances it even caused death from dehydration in young athletes. Yet, I often see 40- to 60-year-olds doggedly avoiding water during tennis matches played in the middle of the day in hot summer weather.

Imagine trying to run your business with information that is 25 years out of date. Not a good idea unless you're in the antiques business.

While some principles never change, much of the fitness and nutrition information on which executives depend is at least 25 years out of date, and, worse, typically designed for an 18- to 25-year-old body rather than a 45- to 65-year-old one.

Major advances in the past decade have led to better understanding of the physiology of exercise and how it relates to health and fitness. Here are seven basic steps, with exercise prescriptions at three levels, to help you start or improve your health and fitness program.

1. Make a Commitment to Total Fitness

The jogging and running boom that exploded in the 1970s and early 1980s introduced a whole generation of executives to the multiple benefits of aerobic conditioning. Previously sedentary executives learned that they not only had more energy and could get more done when they exercised regularly but also felt better and looked healthier.

As the running/jogging movement matured, exercisers learned that aerobic conditioning, while very important, does not provide all of the most important fitness benefits by itself. Nothing drove this point home more dramatically than the untimely death of running enthusiast and author Jim Fixx, who was regarded by many as the "high priest" of the running movement. Throughout his early adult years, Fixx had led a sedentary existence, eaten a diet laden with cholesterol, and allowed his weight to balloon to 240 or 250 pounds. Once he discovered running, he turned his life around. In his books, Fixx talked about running as his medicine and extolled its virtues.

Unfortunately, the same enthusiasm that enlivened his writing may have contributed to his death. During the last few months of his life, he ignored symptoms of increased shortness of breath and occasional chest discomfort, apparently assuming that his running protected him from coronary heart disease. He was 52 years old when he dropped dead running on a country road in Vermont.

Fixx's death sent shock waves through the exercise community. Unfortunately, many people drew the wrong inference that exercise was dangerous and used it as an excuse to remain sedentary. If there is a silver lining in this tragedy, however, it is the reiteration that one component of a fitness program practiced alone is not enough. Aerobic exercise represents a good start, but it must be combined with other elements such as good nutrition, risk factor reduction, and stress control.

2. Check Your Health: Do You Need a Physical?

If you are already actively involved in a fitness program—particularly an exercise routine—there is no need to see your physician. Simply use the self-tests in this chapter as a guide to your level of fitness. If, however, you have been sedentary and not following an overall fitness program, see your physician first for a complete physical examination and a few simple tests. The evaluation should include a history, physical exam (with particular emphasis on the cardiovascular system), resting electrocardiogram, and a blood sample drawn for cholesterol level.

Executives often wonder if they should also undergo a "stress" test—in medical parlance, a graded exercise tolerance test (ETT). What are the guidelines? Such a test is a common part of many physical exams and assessments. In fact, 63% of the executives in our survey reported that they had undergone an ETT. The test generates two types of information. First, it plays a diagnostic role. While you walk or run on a treadmill at progressively faster speeds and steeper inclines, your physician can check your electrocardiogram for signs of ischemia (inadequate blood flow to the heart). Thus, the test can be used as a screening when coronary heart disease (CHD) is suspected.

The second piece of information from an ETT is exercise capacity. How long you can exercise in a standardized format and the maximum heart rate you achieve are both critical guidelines for establishing your exercise prescription.

The confusion about who should undergo a stress test is compounded by physicians who advocate its use as a screening device for most adults. The problem with using the ETT as a generalized screening device to detect CHD in individuals with no symptoms of this problem (for example, no chest pain or shortness of breath with exercise) is that it is more likely to yield a false positive test than a true positive test. Even in an individual who has a worrisome symptom, the ETT can raise a false alarm if not properly performed and interpreted. Consider, for example, the investment banker who went to his physician for a checkup. He was 45 and wanted to become more active in a fitness program, so his doctor recommended an ETT.

Since this particular individual had a very hard-driving and impatient personality, he insisted that the technician start the treadmill at a fairly high speed. He then just jumped on the treadmill. He ran for several minutes at this speed before becoming exhausted, and the test was stopped. Unfortunately, his electrocardiogram showed some worrisome changes, and the banker insisted on an immediate heart catheterization—which showed normal coronary arteries.

Two mistakes had been made. First, the banker should never have been allowed to jump on the treadmill without warming up. Sudden, strenuous exercise is not only dangerous but also can increase the likelihood of the false positive results that occurred in this case. Second, since the patient had no symptoms of heart disease and no risk factors, the next test should have been a thallium ETT, which is more sensitive and specific than a regular ETT. The heart catheterization, which is an invasive procedure that creates discomfort and risk, should have been used only as a last resort.

If an individual has symptoms of CHD, such as chest discomfort with exertion, the argument is entirely different and an ETT is an excellent screening device to suggest whether or not heart disease is present.

As a tool for guiding exercise prescription, the ETT is well established. Both the American Heart Association and the American College of Sports Medicine recommend that previously sedentary individuals over age 45 undergo an ETT prior to starting a new exercise program. The results are particularly useful to quantify the level of exercise and gauge progress over time.

Individuals with significant risk factor for CHD—particularly those who smoke or have high cholesterol or elevated blood pressure—should undergo this test at an earlier age, and certainly if they are over 35.

If you have the test, it should be done in a laboratory that has extensive experience with the procedure. A physician should be in attendance—preferably a cardiologist. I see all too many patients with misleading or incomplete information because the ETT was not properly performed.

3. Learn Your Target Training Zone

One skill to acquire before you start any exercise program is learning to determine your target heart rate or "target training zone." This is a predetermined level of intensity, in heartbeats per minute, to aim for as you exercise. It will ensure maximum aerobic benefits for your efforts. Monitoring your heart rate is the best way to tell if you are exercising at the proper level, or if you should slow down or speed up.

The easiest way to take your pulse is to feel it at the artery on one wrist with the fingertips (but not the thumb) of the other hand. Count the number of beats you feel for 15 seconds, and then multiply by 4 to establish the number of beats per minute. For example, if you count 18 beats in 15 seconds when you are sitting calmly at your desk, your resting heart rate is 72 (18 × 4) beats per minute.

Your target training zone is a percentage of your predicted *maximum* heart rate. To some extent, maximum heart rate is genetically determined. However, it is consistent enough among different individuals so that some simple rules can be used to estimate it. We also know that maximum heart rate decreases with age. Thus, the maximum achievable heart rate of a 55-year-old is significantly less than that of a 25-year-old. (Yet another reason not to gear your exercise with information taught to you in college or by "the old coach.")

To calculate your target zone, follow these simple steps:

1. Determine your predicted maximum heart rate: Subtract your age in years from 220. If you are 55, for example, your predicted maximum heart rate is 165 beats per minute ($220 - 55 = 165$).
2. Multiply your maximum heart rate by the percentage you intend to use for your workouts. A 55-year-old, previously sedentary executive, for example, might start an exercise program with a target of 60% to 70% of his or her maximum predicted heart rate. If that rate is 165, then the target training zone for starting workouts would be 99 to 116 beats per minute ($165 \times .60 = 99$; $165 \times .70 = 116$).

The target training zone that you should use depends on your own goals. Olympic athletes often train at 80% to 90% of their predicted maximum heart rates. That is much too high for the average individual seeking an improved fitness level. The appropriate target zone for improved overall fitness is 60% to 80% of your predicted maximum heart rate. The starter workouts later in this chapter are geared to the lower side of this range (60% to 70%), while the average and expert programs are on the upper side (up to 80%).

How often should you take your pulse? If you are starting a new exercise program I usually recommend that you take your pulse three minutes after you start the training portion of your workout and every five minutes thereafter. Once you have established a routine you can take your pulse less frequently. Often experienced exercisers take their pulse about five minutes into the workout and then toward the end of the workout.

4. Start Slowly and Build Up

Executives often underestimate how long they have been away from exercise. The resulting rush to get in shape often results in sore muscles, discouragement, and even potentially serious injury. The short-term training benefits of exercise, while highly relevant to the executive, are not the key reason to participate in regular exercise. The most important cardiovascular health benefits come from consistent, lifelong exercise. So take it easy when you start and proceed gradually to increase your exercise level.

While eventually you will want to exercise at a level that results in training benefits, don't worry about it at first. It's much more important to devise a program that you enjoy, feel comfortable with, and are likely to stay with throughout your life. Aerobic exercise is a classic example of a race that is truly won by the tortoise rather than the hare.

From the very beginning, make it a habit to warm up before you exercise and cool down afterward. Failure to warm up and cool down will make your exercise uncomfortable, at the very least. And in the worst case, you will expose yourself to potential cardiovascular dangers or orthopedic injury by ignoring before-and-after conditioning. In my experience, the cool-down is most frequently skipped—a bad habit since cooling down and stretching at the end of exercise helps your body improve its flexibility and rid the muscles of waste. Your muscles and tendons are warmed up immediately following exercise—a perfect time to stretch them. Just as important, a gentle cool-down of 5 to 10 minutes allows the heart to gradually decelerate, minimizing the risk of heart rhythm problems.

Finally, before you begin an exercise program, know your starting fitness level. Besides ensuring that you begin with the appropriate amount of exercise, this will provide a bench mark for measuring your progress. Even if you're an experienced exerciser, it's important to know your fitness level so you can check yourself periodically. Later in this chapter, you will find simple tests you can administer yourself, or have an exercise specialist perform for you, to determine your fitness level for aerobic, muscular, and flexibility training.

5. Make Aerobic Exercise the Cornerstone

Aerobic exercise is clearly the best type of exercise for your cardiovascular system, both in terms of short-term fitness benefits and long-term health improvements. I am all in favor of competitive sports such as golf, tennis, or downhill skiing, but alone they are not enough to achieve the most important cardiovascular benefits. Some sports, such as basketball or soccer, have large aerobic components since the running they require is almost continuous; however, when there are periods of stopping and standing around (for example, on the company softball team), the aerobic benefits decline quickly.

Base your fitness program on aerobic conditioning and add other activities to this solid core. In practice, the best aerobic exercises use large muscle groups repetitively for at least 20 to 30 minutes. These exercises include jogging, walking, swimming, cycling (stationary or bicycle), rowing, cross-country skiing, and aerobic dance.

The first step toward this all-important building block—aerobic conditioning—is to estimate your aerobic capacity (known as VO_2 max, or maximum volume of oxygen consumed). There are a number of ways to do it. Historically, the most widely used test was the Harvard Step Test, which required stepping up and down onto a bench for a predetermined number of times during a 3-minute exercise period. The heart rate response was then measured. Subsequent tests involved stationary cycling, running a mile and a half, and determining how far you could run in 12 minutes.

All of these tests had significant limitations. Over the past three years, researchers at our exercise physiology laboratory have developed a simple, highly accurate test for estimating aerobic capacity which only requires that you walk a mile briskly and record your time and heart rate at the end of the walk. The test is called the Rockport Fitness Walking Test ©, after the company that sponsored the research. To take the test you need a measured mile. Most high schools have measured quarter-mile tracks, or you can measure out a mile near your home. The only requirements are that the route be fairly flat with no interruptions (that is, no stop lights or major intersections).

To take the test, wear loose clothing and your favorite walking shoes. Be sure to properly stretch and warm up for 5 to 10 minutes before walking the mile. Walk it as briskly as you can, maintaining a steady pace. At the end of the mile, note the time it took you to walk the mile and your heart rate at the end of the test. Your heart rate should be taken *immediately* at the end of the test. Simply palpate the pulse at your wrist, count the number of beats in 15 seconds, and multiply by 4 to get your exercise heart rate in beats per minute. With this information, turn to the series of charts in figure 1. Find the right chart for your age and sex. Draw a vertical line from your time to walk the mile and a horizontal line from your heart rate. Where the lines cross indicates your fitness level compared with that of other individuals of your age and sex. These fitness levels are based on norms established by the American Heart Association.

If you have undergone an ETT, at your health club or physician's

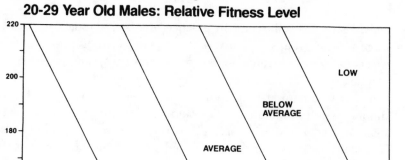

20-29 Year Old Males: Relative Fitness Level

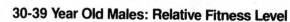

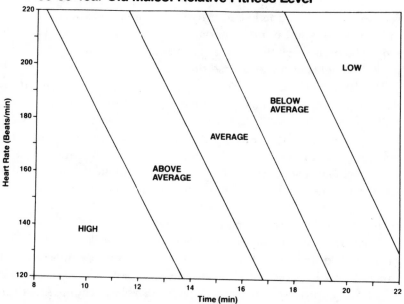

30-39 Year Old Males: Relative Fitness Level

40-49 Year Old Males: Relative Fitness Level

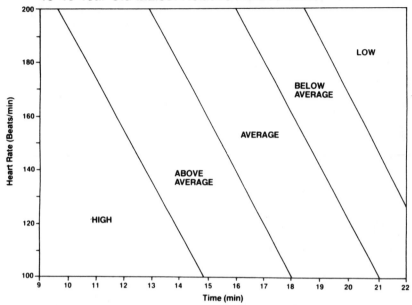

50-59 Year Old Males: Relative Fitness Level

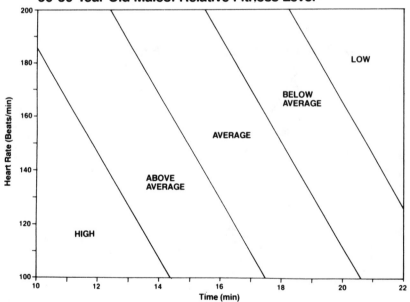

*VO$_2$ norms established by the American Heart Association "Exercise Testing and Training of apparently healthy individuals: A handbook for physicians," Albert A. Kattus, M.D., et al. American Heart Association, New York, 1972.

No exercise test or program should be undertaken without the consent of your personal physician.

60 and over Males: Relative Fitness Level

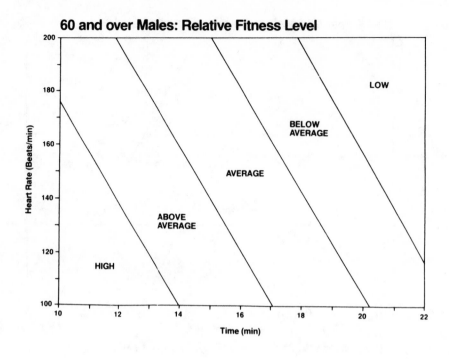

20-29 Year Old Females: Relative Fitness Level

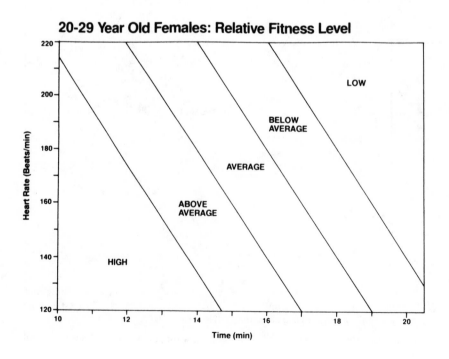

30-39 Year Old Females: Relative Fitness Level

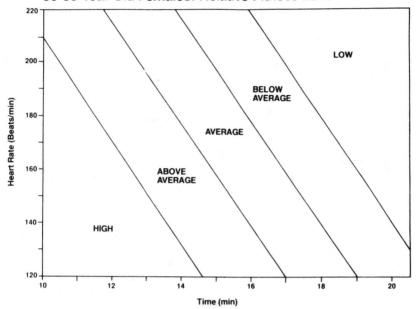

40-49 Year Old Females: Relative Fitness Level

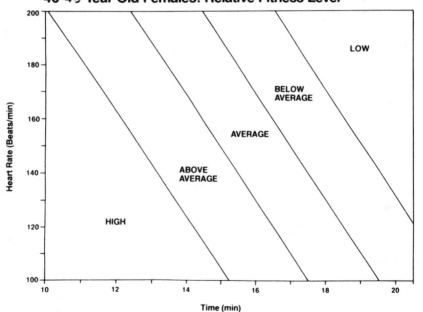

43

50-59 Year Old Females: Relative Fitness Level

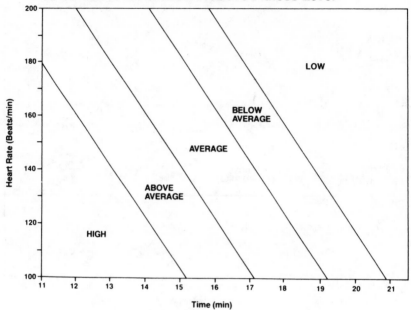

60 and over Females: Relative Fitness Level

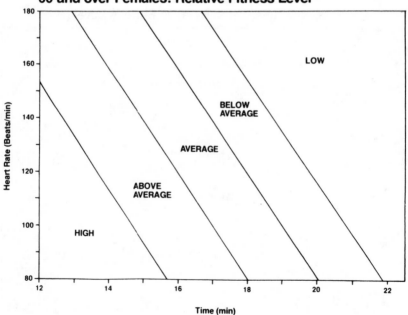

office, for example, your performance can be used to estimate your aerobic capacity. If the test you took employed a standard "Bruce Protocol" (a particular exercise protocol named after its inventor, Dr. Robert Bruce—used by about 90% of hospitals), simply use the number of minutes and seconds you walked or ran on the test and plug them into the Foster equations below to get an estimate of your aerobic capacity.

$$VO_2 \text{ max} = 14.8 - 1.379 \text{ (TIME)} + 0.451 \text{ (TIME}^2) - 0.012 \text{ (TIME}^3)$$

TIME = number of minutes on the treadmill to the nearest minute.

Once you have pinpointed your current aerobic capacity, you will know your fitness level and where to begin your program—at the starter, average, or expert stage. These aerobic capacity tests tell you your current level of cardiovascular fitness. They are not *diagnostic* tests in the sense that they are not designed to screen whether or not you have CHD; however, the aerobic capacity tests do tell you how your current fitness stacks up against that of other individuals of your age and sex. They also give you a bench mark against which to gauge progress as you get in better shape. With the latest information on the major aerobic exercises as background, here are three different levels of programs for the five most popular activities: jogging, walking, swimming, cycling, and rowing.

If you scored in the "low" or "below average" category on the Rockport Fitness Walking Test or had a VO_2 max of less than 30 on the Foster equations, you should start with the starter program of aerobic exercise. If you scored in the "average" or "above average" category on the Rockport Fitness Walking Test or between 30 and 45 on the Foster equations, start with the average program of aerobic conditioning. If you scored in the "high" category on the Rockport Fitness Walking Test or above 45 on the Foster equations, start with the expert program of aerobic conditioning.

Jogging

No other exercise for aerobic conditioning has had greater impact on American executives during the past 15 years than jogging. It was the fitness activity most frequently listed by respondents to our survey, with 23% indicating that they regularly—at least three times a week—jog or run. Some of the most animated conversations I've had with executives involved their jogging programs. Like Tenneco's J. L. Ketelsen, many cited favorite runs in exotic business locations in addition to their normal routines when at home. Some even related stories of competitive running achievements.

"The most exciting run I've ever had was the Houston Marathon," noted K. W. Reese, pointing to a picture in his office of four Tenneco executives (including himself) running in the marathon. "I can't describe what it was like. Here's a guy who had had open heart surgery—Ketelsen—and another one, who had had a heart attack, running along with these two other guys on this beautiful day in Houston. I turned to Ketelsen and said, 'You know, it's been thirty-five years since I've been on Main Street before a crowd with a band playing. And that was in 1952, after we beat Baylor thirty-seven to seven!'" "So it was like being a kid again," Reese continued, "—like we beat Baylor again that day and we're running up the middle of Main Street to the cheers of the crowd."

There is no question that jogging or running is an excellent activity for cardiovascular conditioning and weight control. Those executives who rely on it, however, also value its psychological benefits, such as stress reduction and sense of higher energy, as equally important reasons for sticking with their programs.

"People who get out and exercise make better workers—they're more mentally alert," observed Ciprico's chairman and former president, Ronald Thomas, who once ran a marathon in 3 hours and 16 minutes. "We had a hard core of about ten runners, including a couple from administration, one or two from sales, a few engineers, and a guy in manufacturing. We go out, three or four of us at a time, preferably around noon, and run together. It creates great spirit and we feel good about ourselves."

MCI's Donald Steen, who runs three or four times a week, echoes Thomas's sentiment. "When I don't feel well, I'm not always sure whether it's stress related or lack of exercise," he says. "But it sure helps a lot when I get those running sessions in. When I get out in the morning [to exercise], I plan my whole day. While I'm running, I can think things through and they just become clearer."

Jogging/Running: Starter Program

Week	Exercise	Distance (in miles)	Heart Rate (% of max)	Duration of Workout (min)	Calories Burned*	Frequency (times/wk)
1	Walk/jog	0.5	60–70	8	50	3
2	Walk/jog	0.5	60–70	8	50	3
3	Walk/jog	0.75	60–70	11	75	3
4	Walk/jog	0.75	60–70	11	75	3
5	Walk/jog	1.0	60–70	14	100	3
6	Jog	1.0	70–80	14	100	3
7	Jog	1.25	70–80	16	125	3
8	Jog	1.25	70–80	16	125	3
9	Jog	1.5	70–80	18	150	3
10	Jog	1.5	70–80	18	150	3

*Calories are estimated for a 150-pound individual. If you are heavier, add 10% to the number of calories burned for every 15 pounds above 150. If you weigh less than 150 pounds, subtract 10% from the number of calories burned for every 15 pounds below 150.

MOVING UP: Test yourself after week 10 using the Rockport Fitness Walking Test©. If your test results indicate that you are ready to move up to the next category, you will want to begin at approximately week 5 of the next program.

Jogging/Running: Average Program

Week	Exercise	Distance (in miles)	Heart Rate (% of max)	Duration of Workout (min)	Calories Burned*	Frequency (times/wk)
1	Walk/jog	1.0	60–70	16	100	3
2	Walk/jog	1.0	60–70	16	100	3
3	Walk/jog	1.25	60–70	19	125	3
4	Jog	1.25	70–80	16	125	3
5	Jog	1.5	70–80	18	150	3
6	Jog	1.5	70–80	18	150	3
7	Jog	1.75	70–80	21	175	3
8	Jog	1.75	70–80	21	175	3
9	Jog	2.0	70–80	23	200	3
10	Jog	2.0	70–80	23	200	3

*Calories are estimated for a 150-pound individual. If you are heavier, add 10% to the number of calories burned for every 15 pounds above 150. If you weigh less than 150 pounds, subtract 10% from the number of calories burned for every 15 pounds below 150.

> MOVING UP: Test yourself after week 10 using the Rockport Fitness Walking Test©. If your test results indicate that you are ready to move up to the next category, you will want to begin at approximately week 5 of the next program.

JOGGING/RUNNING: EXPERT PROGRAM

Week	Exercise	Distance (in miles)	Heart Rate (% of max)	Duration of Workout (min)	Calories Burned*	Frequency (times/wk)
1	Jog	2.0	70–80	20	200	3
2	Jog	2.0	70–80	18	200	3
3	Jog	2.25	70–80	22	225	3
4	Jog	2.25	70–80	20	225	3
5	Jog	2.50	70–80	25	250	3
6	Jog	2.50	70–80	23	250	3
7	Jog	2.75	70–80	27	275	3
8	Jog	2.75	70–80	25	275	3
9	Jog	3.0	70–80	30	300	3
10	Jog	3.0	70–80	27	300	3

*Calories are estimated for a 150-pound individual. If you are heavier, add 10% to the number of calories burned for every 15 pounds above 150. If you weigh less than 150 pounds, subtract 10% from the number of calories burned for every 15 pounds below 150.

Once you have reached week 10 of the expert program you are ready for a lifelong maintenance program.

> MAINTENANCE PROGRAM: Warm up and stretch 5–7 minutes; jog 3.0 miles at a pace of 9 minutes/mile (approximately 6.5 mph); cool down and stretch for 5–7 minutes.

Once you have completed the 10-week initial exercise program, retest yourself with the Rockport Fitness Walking Test© to establish a new level of exercise program. After you complete the 10 weeks of the expert program, proceed to the maintenance program for lifelong fitness.

Although jogging is an excellent aerobic activity for many individuals, you need to be cautious if you have a history of any orthopedic problem. Remember, when you jog you actually leave the ground on every stride. When you land, you exert forces equal to three to four times your body weight each time your foot hits the ground. This can aggravate a previous orthopedic injury or weakness or cause one if you have been sedentary or are significantly overweight.

Fitness Walking

Many experts believe that fitness walking will be the major adult fitness activity in the United States for the next 20 years. There are already a number of studies that support this conclusion. A 1987 survey by the National Sporting Goods Association estimated that 54 million Americans were exercise walkers, compared with 23 million joggers and 18 million swimmers. Major market research organizations, including Gallup and American Sports Data, Inc., have conducted studies showing that the major growth in exercise programs in the United States comes primarily from individuals adopting walking programs.

In our survey, 20% of the executives listed fitness walking as a regular activity, a figure that I suspect is considerably less than the actual number who walk but don't classify it as a separate exercise activity. Our Exercise Physiology Laboratory at UMass Medical School has been particularly interested in fitness walking for the past five years and, with other scientific and medical researchers, has uncovered significant new information about walking's cardiovascular benefits.

The efficacy of fitness walking as an aerobic training exercise has been vastly underestimated in the past. In studies in our laboratory of more than 600 people between the ages of 20 and 79, more than 90% of women and 67% of men—regardless of age or previous level of conditioning—were able to elevate their heart rate into the target training zone with brisk walking. The speeds to accomplish this were not particularly fast, averaging 4.1 miles per hour (mph), or only 33% higher than the average walking speed of 3 mph. To put this in perspective, most people need only reach a speed that they would regard as "determined" walking to derive training benefits from fitness walking.

Walking is also an excellent activity for weight loss—probably the preferred way to lose weight. The average 150-pound person burns approximately 100 calories walking a mile. People are often surprised to learn that if they take a brisk 45-minute walk four times a week for a year and don't increase the amount of food they eat, they will burn enough calories to lose 18 pounds. More important, virtually all of the weight lost will be fat because regular exercise preserves lean muscle mass.

Besides aerobic and weight control benefits, however, fitness walking offers a key advantage most other exercises do not: lifetime application. In short, you can keep it up. Most of the research linking exercise to cardiovascular health emphasizes that lifelong consistency appears to be more important than intensity. In the College Alumni Study of more than 16,000 college graduates, for example, those who reported consistent physical activity were significantly less likely to develop coronary heart disease than their more sedentary counterparts.

One aspect of fitness walking that makes it particularly favorable for lifetime exercise is the low injury potential. When you jog, you leave the ground with each stride. When you land, the forces on the bones and joints are typically 3 to 4 times your body weight. In walking, however, one foot is always on the ground. Thus, the impact forces per stride are considerably less—typically 1 to 1.25 times your body weight.

As with all of the aerobic exercise programs, determine where to start by taking the Rockport Fitness Walking Test©. Retest yourself with the Rockport Fitness Walking Test© after 10 weeks of fitness walking. This will help you determine if you are ready to move up to the next fitness category. When you move up, you will typically start at about week 5 of the next fitness category.

FITNESS WALKING: STARTER PROGRAM

Week	Distance (in miles)	Pace* (mph)	Heart Rate (% of max)	Duration of Workout (min)	Calories Burned†	Frequency (times/wk)
1	0.5	3.0	60–70	10	50	3
2	0.5	3.0	60–70	10	50	3
3	0.75	3.5	60–70	13	75	3
4	0.75	3.5	60–70	13	75	3
5	1.0	3.5	60–70	17	100	3
6	1.0	3.5	60–70	17	100	3
7	1.25	4.0	70–80	19	125	3
8	1.25	4.0	70–80	19	125	3
9	1.5	4.5	70–80	20	150	3
10	1.5	4.5	70–80	20	150	3

*Pace is approximate. Actual exercise should be geared to maintain heart rate at designated percentage of maximum.
†Calories burned are estimated for a 150-pound person.

> MOVING UP: Test yourself after week 10 using the Rockport Fitness Walking Test©. If your test results indicate that you are ready to move up to the next category, you will want to begin at approximately week 5 of the next program.

FITNESS WALKING: AVERAGE PROGRAM

Week	Distance (in miles)	Pace* (mph)	Heart Rate (% of max)	Duration of Workout (min)	Calories Burned†	Frequency (times/wk)
1	1.0	3.0	60–70	20	100	3
2	1.0	3.0	60–70	20	100	3
3	1.25	3.5	60–70	21	125	3
4	1.25	3.5	60–70	21	125	3
5	1.50	3.5	60–70	26	150	3
6	1.50	3.5	60–70	26	150	3
7	1.75	4.0	70–80	26	175	3
8	1.75	4.0	70–80	26	175	3
9	2.0	4.5	70–80	26	200	3
10	2.0	4.5	70–80	26	200	3

*Pace is approximate. Actual exercise should be geared to maintain heart rate at designated percentage of maximum.
†Calories burned are estimated for a 150-pound person.

> MOVING UP: Test yourself after week 10 using the Rockport Fitness
> Walking Test©. If your test results indicate that you are
> ready to move up to the next category, you will want to begin
> at approximately week 5 of the next program.

FITNESS WALKING: EXPERT PROGRAM

Week	Distance (in miles)	Pace* (mph)	Heart Rate (% of max)	Duration of Workout (min)	Calories Burned†	Frequency (times/wk)
1	2.0	4.0	70–80	30	200	3
2	2.0	4.0	70–80	30	200	3
3	2.25	4.0	70–80	34	225	3
4	2.25	4.0	70–80	34	225	3
5	2.50	4.0	70–80	38	250	3
6	2.50	4.5	70–80	33	250	3
7	2.75	4.5	70–80	37	275	3
8	2.75	4.5	70–80	37	275	3
9	3.0	4.5	70–80	40	300	3
10	3.0	4.5	70–80	40	300	3

*Pace is approximate. Actual exercise should be geared to maintain heart rate at designated percentage of maximum.

†Calories burned are estimated for a 150-pound person.

By the time you have reached week 10 of the expert program, you are ready to think about a lifelong maintenance program. Several good ways to add variety to your walking program are to add hills or light hand weights. The hand weights should be pumped up and down as you walk, with a controlled motion from hip to shoulder height. One good, and often ignored, way to add hills to your workout is to climb some stairs at the beginning or end.

> MAINTENANCE PROGRAM: Warm up and stretch for 5–7 minutes; fitness
> walk 3.0 miles at a 4.5-mph pace; cool down
> and stretch for 5–7 minutes.

Swimming

This is one of the great total body conditioners, but far fewer executives swim regularly than walk, jog, or cycle. Only 9% of the survey respondents listed swimming as a regular fitness activity, yet, as an exercise, it has several important advantages.

First, because the water supports your weight, swimming puts virtually no stress on bones and joints. This makes it an ideal activity for individuals with joint problems. Second, in virtually every different type of swimming stroke, more power comes from the upper body than from the legs. In the crawl stroke, for example, about 70% of the power comes from the arms and 30% from the legs. This makes swimming an ideal way to build upper body strength and endurance.

The major drawbacks of swimming are obvious: It takes special facilities and you need reasonable skill levels to make it your primary form of fitness activity. In my experience, most executives simply lack the swimming skill to make it their main activity and consider the inconvenience of going to a pool a major problem.

SWIMMING: STARTER PROGRAM

Week	Distance* (in yards)	Heart Rate† (% of max)	Calories Burned‡	Frequency (times/wk)
1	200	60–70	42	3
2	250	60–70	52	3
3	300	60–70	64	3
4	350	60–70	74	3
5	400	60–70	84	3
6	450	70–80	94	3
7	500	70–80	106	3
8	550	70–80	116	3
9	600	70–80	127	3
10	700	70–80	148	3

*Rest 30 seconds after every 50 yards.

†The heart rate should be determined during one of your 30-second rest periods. Determine the heart rate by feeling the pulse at your wrist as already described. Do this as quickly as possible after reaching the end of the pool.

‡Assumes a 150-pound person swimming at 50 yards per minute.

MOVING UP: Test yourself after week 10 using the Rockport Fitness Walking Test©. If your test results indicate that you are ready to move up to the next category, you will want to begin at approximately week 5 of the next program.

SWIMMING: AVERAGE PROGRAM

Week	Distance* (in yards)	Heart Rate† (% of max)	Calories Burned‡	Frequency (times/wk)
1	500	60–70	106	3
2	550	60–70	116	3
3	600	60–70	127	3
4	650	60–70	137	3
5	700	60–70	148	3
6	750	70–80	158	3
7	800	70–80	168	3
8	850	70–80	178	3
9	900	70–80	189	3
10	1000	70–80	210	3

*Rest 30 seconds after every 50 yards.

†The heart rate should be determined during one of your 30-second rest periods. Determine the heart rate by feeling the pulse at your wrist as already described. Do this as quickly as possible after reaching the end of the pool.

‡Assumes a 150-pound person swimming at 50 yards per minute.

> MOVING UP: Test yourself after week 10 using the Rockport Fitness Walking Test©. If your test results indicate that you are ready to move up to the next category, you will want to begin at approximately week 5 of the next program.

SWIMMING: EXPERT PROGRAM

Week	Distance* (in yards)	Heart Rate† (% of max)	Calories Burned‡	Frequency (times/wk)
1	800	70–80	168	3
2	850	70–80	178	3
3	900	70–80	189	3
4	950	70–80	200	3
5	1000	70–80	210	3
6	1050	70–80	221	3
7	1100	70–80	231	3
8	1150	70–80	241	3
9	1200	70–80	252	3
10	1300	70–80	274	3

*Rest 30 seconds after every 50 yards.

†The heart rate should be determined during one of your 30-second rest periods. Determine the heart rate by feeling the pulse at your wrist as already described. Do this as quickly as possible after reaching the end of the pool.

‡Assumes a 150-pound person swimming at 50 yards per minute.

Once you have reached week 10 of the expert program, you are ready for a lifelong maintenance program.

MAINTENANCE PROGRAM:	Warm up and stretch for 5–7 minutes; swim 1,300 yards, maintaining a heart rate of 70–80% of predicted maximum; cool down and stretch for 5–7 minutes.

Cycling

Indoor stationary cycling and outdoor recreational cycling are excellent aerobic conditioners. When statistics for the two are combined, the number of executives who cycle is equal to the number who fitness walk or jog. Within the cycling category, however, stationary pedaling is three times more popular as regular exercise than outdoor pedaling (17% of respondents versus 6%).

Besides being an excellent conditioner, cycling offers the considerable advantage of placing virtually no impact on the bones or joints. It's also excellent for weight loss. In a 30-minute workout, you can burn between 200 and 300 calories. Numerous studies on the physiology of stationary cycling have concluded that, for most people, it provides a better mode of cardiovascular conditioning than outdoor cycling. There are several reasons.

Most recreational cyclists lack the skills that would allow them to go fast enough to achieve cardiovascular training benefits without significant danger to life and limb. Furthermore, in most urban and suburban environments, traffic and cross streets make cycling very much a stop-and-go proposition. This should not be construed as an indictment of outdoor cycling, which is a superb cardiovascular conditioner. Some of the top amateur cyclists we have studied in our exercise physiology laboratory have had cardiovascular levels that rank among the top of all athletes we have measured. The simple reality is that most executives are not highly skilled cyclists, nor do they live in areas conducive to unimpeded, high-speed cycling. For them, stationary cycling is a much more realistic cardiovascular conditioning activity.

Many executives use stationary cycling as one alternative among several aerobic exercises in their overall programs. Having their own cycle gives them the option of working out at their convenience and, particularly, during inclement weather. With recent advances in technology,

55

there are now excellent, computer-enhanced stationary cycles that inter-act with the user and minimize the boredom many executives complain about.

Among the proponents of stationary cycling is NASA scientist and Interand Corporation CEO Leonard Reiffel, who suddenly realized one day that "I was getting too fat and too old and just didn't want that to happen." His solution evolved from a combination of stationary cycling, rowing, lifting free weights, and occasional light jogging. "I cycle about half an hour a day, five or six days a week," Reiffel reported. "Boredom? You can beat it. My setup includes a TV set, and I recently added a reading stand that I equipped with very strong magnets taken from the latest NMR [nuclear magnetic resonance] technology. The magnets hold down the pages of whatever I'm reading." The exercise program also has held down his weight, toned up his body, and reduced his blood pressure to 120/78.

STATIONARY CYCLING: STARTER PROGRAM

Week	RPM	Heart Rate* (% of max)	Duration of Workout (min)	Calories Burned†	Frequency (times/wk)
1	60–80	60–70	10	58	3
2	60–80	60–70	10	58	3
3	60–80	60–70	12	68	3
4	60–80	60–70	14	80	3
5	60–80	60–70	16	91	3
6	60–80	70–80	16	91	3
7	60–80	70–80	18	103	3
8	60–80	70–80	18	103	3
9	60–80	70–80	20	114	3
10	60–80	70–80	20	114	3

*Determine heart rate by palpating the artery at one wrist using the fingertips of the other hand. Set the intensity of resistance on your stationary cycle to maintain the percentage of maximum heart rate indicated.

†Calories burned are based on a 150-pound individual pedaling at the RPM and percentage of maximum heart rate indicated.

MOVING UP: Test yourself after week 10 using the Rockport Fitness Walking Test©. If your test results indicate that you are ready to move up to the next category, you will want to begin at approximately week 5 of the next program.

STATIONARY CYCLING: AVERAGE PROGRAM

Week	RPM	Heart Rate* (% of max)	Duration of Workout (min)	Calories Burned†	Frequency (times/wk)
1	60–80	60–70	15	86	3
2	60–80	60–70	15	86	3
3	60–80	60–70	18	103	3
4	60–80	60–70	18	103	3
5	60–80	60–70	20	114	3
6	60–80	70–80	20	114	3
7	60–80	70–80	23	131	3
8	60–80	70–80	23	131	3
9	60–80	70–80	25	143	3
10	60–80	70–80	25	143	3

*Determine heart rate by palpating the artery at one wrist using the fingertips of the other hand. Set the intensity of resistance on your stationary cycle to maintain the percentage of maximum heart rate indicated.

†Calories burned are based on a 150-pound individual pedaling at the RPM and percentage of maximum heart rate indicated.

MOVING UP: Test yourself after week 10 using the Rockport Fitness Walking Test©. If your test results indicate that you are ready to move up to the next category, you will want to begin at approximately week 5 of the next program.

STATIONARY CYCLING: EXPERT PROGRAM

Week	RPM	Heart Rate* (% of max)	Duration of Workout (min)	Calories Burned†	Frequency (times/wk)
1	60–80	70–80	20	114	3
2	60–80	70–80	22	125	3
3	60–80	70–80	24	137	3
4	60–80	70–80	24	137	3
5	60–80	70–80	26	148	3
6	60–80	70–80	26	148	3
7	60–80	70–80	28	160	3
8	60–80	70–80	28	160	3
9	60–80	70–80	30	172	3
10	60–80	70–80	30	172	3

*Determine heart rate by palpating the artery at one wrist using the fingertips of the other hand. Set the intensity of resistance on your stationary cycle to maintain the percentage of maximum heart rate indicated.

†Calories burned are based on a 150-pound individual pedaling at the RPM and percentage of maximum heart rate indicated.

Once you have reached week 10 of the expert program, you are ready for a lifelong maintenance program.

> MAINTENANCE PROGRAM: Warm up and stretch for 5–7 minutes; cycle for 30 minutes at heart rate of 70–80% of predicted maximum; cool down and stretch for 5–7 minutes.

Rowing

As a form of aerobic conditioning and total body exercise, rowing rivals swimming. But, again, there is the substantial drawback of the need for specialized equipment and facilities. New developments in stationary rowing machines for home use are circumventing this problem. Still, only 3% of the executives responding to our survey indicated rowing as one of their regular forms of exercise.

Rowing is not only an excellent cardiovascular conditioner but also an excellent way to build abdominal, back, and leg muscle strength. As for weight control, a 30-minute workout on a rowing machine will burn an average of 250 to 400 calories, depending on your fitness level.

The best types of indoor machines are those that closely duplicate the motion you would use if you were sculling on a river or lake. Models that require you to bend over at the beginning of a stroke are not as good since they may cause back strain. To reduce the boredom factor, new computer-enhanced models provide colorful graphics.

Among the executives who extolled the virtues of rowing, none was more enthusiastic than William Coors, of Adolph Coors Company, who rows seven days a week. "I was a jogger until I developed a problem on the left side of my knee," he recalled. "It ended my running and skiing. I tried fast walking on a treadmill, but it was too close to running, which I wasn't supposed to be doing. So I got a rowing machine—and, in the process, discovered as complete an exercise as you can get."

ROWING: STARTER PROGRAM

Week	Strokes per Minute	Heart Rate (% of max)	Duration of Workout (min)	Calories Burned*	Frequency (times/wk)
1	26–28	60–70	10	100	3
2	26–28	60–70	10	100	3
3	26–28	60–70	12	120	3
4	26–28	60–70	14	140	3
5	26–28	60–70	16	160	3
6	28–30	70–80	16	160	3
7	28–30	70–80	18	180	3
8	28–30	70–80	18	180	3
9	28–30	70–80	20	200	3
10	28–30	70–80	20	200	3

*Based on a 150-pound individual rowing at a moderate intensity and burning 10 calories per minute. Actual calories burned depends on the level of resistance on the rowing machine or power used in outdoor rowing.

MOVING UP: Test yourself after week 10 using the Rockport Fitness Walking Test©. If your test results indicate that you are ready to move up to the next category, you will want to begin at approximately week 5 of the next program.

ROWING: AVERAGE PROGRAM

Week	Strokes per Minute	Heart Rate (% of max)	Duration of Workout (min)	Calories Burned*	Frequency (times/wk)
1	28–30	60–70	15	150	3
2	28–30	60–70	15	150	3
3	28–30	60–70	18	180	3
4	28–30	60–70	18	180	3
5	28–30	60–70	20	200	3
6	30–32	70–80	20	200	3
7	30–32	70–80	23	230	3
8	30–32	70–80	23	230	3
9	30–32	70–80	25	250	3
10	30–32	70–80	25	250	3

*Based on a 150-pound individual rowing at a moderate intensity and burning 10 calories per minute. Actual calories burned depends on the level of resistance on the rowing machine or power used in outdoor rowing.

MOVING UP: Test yourself after week 10 using the Rockport Fitness Walking Test©. If your test results indicate that you are ready to move up to the next category, you will want to begin at approximately week 5 of the next program.

ROWING: EXPERT PROGRAM

Week	Strokes per Minute	Heart Rate (% of max)	Duration of Workout (min)	Calories Burned*	Frequency (times/wk)
1	30–32	70–80	20	200	3
2	30–32	70–80	22	220	3
3	30–32	70–80	24	240	3
4	30–32	70–80	24	240	3
5	30–32	70–80	26	260	3
6	34–36	70–80	26	260	3
7	34–36	70–80	28	280	3
8	34–36	70–80	28	280	3
9	34–36	70–80	30	300	3
10	34–36	70–80	30	300	3

*Based on a 150-pound individual rowing at a moderate intensity and burning 10 calories per minute. Actual calories burned depends on the level of resistance on the rowing machine or power used in outdoor rowing.

Once you have reached week 10 of the expert program, you are ready for a lifelong maintenance program.

MAINTENANCE PROGRAM: Warm up and stretch for 5–7 minutes; row for 30 minutes at heart rate of 70–80% of predicted maximum; cool down and stretch for 5–7 minutes.

6. Add Strength Training

Aerobic exercise is not the only form of exercise you should pursue. I typically start executives on high-repetition, low-weight musculoskeletal strength training in conjunction with aerobic activity. Musculoskeletal conditioning is an important part of a comprehensive fitness program for a number of reasons.

First, muscular strength and endurance play a key role in preventing injury to the arms, legs, and back. This is particularly important to executives who play tennis, golf, and other sports that require upper body strength and flexibility. I've seen enough executives who have suffered injuries from weekend activities to know that many of the injuries could have been prevented if the individual had had even a minimal ongoing program of muscular conditioning.

There are literally hundreds of different muscular strength and endurance building programs. Couple this with at least 10 different major manufacturers of equipment and it can get pretty confusing. If you keep a couple of simple principles in mind, however, you will have a well-rounded program and accomplish everything you need to.

First, your program should have at least one exercise for each of the major muscle groups. You will see that the program I recommend does just that. The major muscle groups are chest, back, quadriceps, shoulders, hamstrings, abdominals, biceps, calves, triceps, and forearms. Second, establish an order that starts with the largest muscles and works its way out to the smallest muscles. It is also a good idea to have a sequence that alternates trunk, upper body, and lower body. In other words, don't do all your upper-body exercises one right after the other, followed by all your lower-body exercises.

Regular musculoskeletal conditioning can also lessen back problems. One CEO noted that if he walked out of his office and shouted, "I've found the cure for low back pain," all executives within hearing range would rush out of their offices to ask about it. Chronic low back pain is often the result of a sedentary life-style that allows the muscles of the back and trunk to become weak.

Muscular strength training is essential to balance aerobic exercise, as many recreational runners have learned the hard way. We first became aware of this in the 1970s when many runners started developing low back pain. Often it was caused by running extended distances regularly without performing any exercises to strengthen and stretch the back. Some of the major leg muscles insert in the lower back and can overpower the back and trunk muscles to create pain. The cure is often to simply add 5 to 10 minutes a day of back and trunk stretching and strengthening.

A final reason for muscular conditioning is toning and appearance. All of the executives I interviewed who are involved in muscular training programs confirmed that the exercises improve the way they look

61

and feel about themselves. Bombarded by images of body builders, many people have the misconception that muscular conditioning is designed for building up large, not very functional, muscles. With the latest approaches to training, however, the emphasis is on building well-toned muscles that will help you in your daily activities, both at work and during recreation.

Interest in weight training among executives is considerable. More than 28% of our survey respondents include some form of strength training as part of their regular exercise routine. Unfortunately, the knowledge concerning musculoskeletal conditioning has not kept pace with the level of interest for most executives. Very few have had the kind of proper instruction that Paul Allaire receives at the Xerox Fitness Center.

"Running is great for my heart and legs, but it doesn't do much for my upper body," noted Allaire. "So I try to use the Nautilus equipment down in the gym two or three times a week. We have a physical therapist who helps us use the weights properly."

Much more common are executives who lift weights based on their high school or college experiences or who have devised their own programs based on little theoretical understanding. Several executives frankly admitted that their weight training was developed through "trial and error." To meld theory and practice properly, it is important to understand the difference between strength, power, and endurance.

Muscular *strength* refers to the maximum amount of weight a muscle can lift for one repetition. Thus, an executive who can lift a 200-pound barbell over his head is twice as strong as one who can lift a 100-pound barbell. Muscular strength alone is not that relevant to the life-styles of most executives, however. Muscular *power* and *endurance* are much more important.

Power is the combination of strength and speed. It is highly relevant to recreational activities since it determines the speed of your first serve in tennis, the length of your drives in golf, or even your ability to survive a morning of expert trails on the ski slopes. Individuals who can drive a golf ball 240 yards consistently have more power in their golf swings than someone who consistently drives 170 yards.

Muscular *endurance* is how many repetitions of an activity a muscle can perform before becoming fatigued. Endurance is highly relevant to how you perform in the third set of a tennis match or the last few holes of a golf game. Endurance also is relevant to how tired you feel at the end of a long day at the office, or how well you function when you get off the plane after a cross-country or transatlantic flight.

There are several easy ways to check your muscular strength and endurance. Two simple do-it-yourself tests are the number of sit-ups you can do in a minute and the total number of push-ups you can do. The sit-ups should be done with your arms crossed in front of your chest. For men the push-ups should be done with your knees off the ground. For women, the push-ups should be done with the knees on the ground and arms extended out slightly further toward the head to provide proper balance. Try to keep back and legs as straight as possible during the push-ups. For the sit-ups, have a friend time you for exactly 60 seconds to see how many you can do. The number of sit-ups will provide an estimate of the strength and endurance of your abdominal muscles; the number of push-ups will give you an estimate of upper body muscular strength and endurance. Here's how to grade yourself:

Sit-ups		Push-ups	
No. Completed in 60 sec.	Strength and Endurance	No. Completed	Strength and Endurance
40 or more	Excellent	40 or more	Excellent
30–39	Good	24–39	Good
20–29	Fair	16–23	Fair
19 or fewer	Poor	15 or fewer	Poor

If you have access to a fitness center or health club, tests of your upper and lower body strength can be performed on various types of weight-training equipment. To test upper body strength, use a bench press; for lower body strength, use the leg press. Both tests should be supervised by a trained exercise specialist. First, determine the maximum amount of weight you can lift with the bench press or leg press (this is a measure of your strength). Then, to determine your upper and lower body endurance, use 70% of the maximum amount you can lift and see how many repetitions of this you can perform.

Since there are so many brands of exercise equipment available, providing universal norms for strength and endurance for the bench press and leg press is virtually impossible. The best advice is to perform these tests under the supervision of the exercise physiologist at your health club and inquire how your results compare to the established norms on the particular equipment used.

Safety in weight training is extremely important. There are a number of steps to keep in mind as you build a program, but none is more important than this: Get proper instruction. Before you start using the exercises outlined here, consult an athletic trainer or exercise specialist at a health club or your corporate fitness center to learn the proper techniques. Trying to set up your own weight-training regimen is an invitation to injury.

The kind of equipment you should use is largely a matter of availability and personal preference. Despite extravagant claims by different manufacturers, most equipment provides similar strength and endurance gains. Free weights, isokinetic equipment, and isotonic equipment are all acceptable. Once again, it is best to check with a local athletic trainer or exercise specialist.

How fast should you progress? The principle of improving strength and endurance is based on the concept of progressive overload—that is, slowly build up the amount of weight lifted and the number of repetitions performed. It takes discipline, however: Don't let your competitive instincts run wild and try to progress too rapidly. Strength gains of 2% to 3% a week are common, a factor you should use as a guideline for how fast to increase the weights as you build your program.

Here are starter, average, and expert programs for conditioning the major muscle groups of the body. These exercises should be performed twice a week with at least a day between sessions, and in the order listed, since they are designed to work the largest muscle groups first.

7. Stay Loose: Keep Stretching

Exercisers and physicians alike have paid too little attention to the role of flexibility—keeping muscles and joints pliable—as a key building block in a comprehensive fitness program. As you follow your aerobic and muscular strength building programs, it's important to include stretching exercises as well. The major reason is to prevent injury.

People often don't realize that while regular exercise builds muscle strength, there is also a tendency for the muscles to become stiffer. This can lead to muscle strain and injury. Even minor soreness that comes from the repetitive use of specific muscle groups can be alleviated by following a proper stretching routine. It is particularly crucial for previously sedentary individuals whose muscles have become smaller and shorter through lack of use. Weak muscles and tendons can result in

MUSCULAR STRENGTH AND ENDURANCE: STARTER AND AVERAGE PROGRAMS

Exercise	Muscles Used	Amount of Weight	Repetitions per Set	Starter (No. of Sets)	Average (No. of Sets)
Bench press	Chest	70% 1 RM*	10	1	2
Bent over rows	Back	70% 1 RM	10	1	2
Quadriceps extension	Quadriceps	70% 1 RM	10	1	2
Upright row	Shoulders	70% 1 RM	10	1	2
Hamstring curls	Hamstrings	70% 1 RM	10	1	2
Sit-ups	Abdominals	†	†	†	†
Biceps curl	Biceps	70% 1 RM	10	1	2
Toe raises with weights on shoulders	Calves	70% 1 RM	10	1	2
Triceps extension	Triceps	70% 1 RM*	10	1	2
Wrist curls	Forearms	70% 1 RM	10	1	2

*1 RM is the maximum amount of weight you can lift for one repetition.
†Start with 70% of the maximum number you can perform in 1 minute.

MUSCULAR STRENGTH AND ENDURANCE: EXPERT PROGRAM

Exercise	Muscles Used	Amount of Weight	Repetitions per Set	No. of Sets
Bench press	Chest	70% 1 RM*	10	3
Bent over rows	Back	70% 1 RM	10	3
Quadriceps extension	Quadriceps	70% 1 RM	10	3
Upright row	Shoulders	70% 1 RM	10	3
Hamstring curls	Hamstrings	70% 1 RM	10	3
Sit-ups	Abdominals	†	†	†
Biceps curl	Biceps	70% 1 RM	10	3
Toe raises with weights on shoulders	Calves	70% 1 RM	10	3
Triceps extension	Triceps	70% 1 RM	10	3
Wrist curls	Forearms	70% 1 RM	10	3

*1 RM is the maximum amount of weight you can lift for one repetition.
†Start with 70% of the maximum number you can perform in 1 minute.

serious injury, such as a tear or pull. Thus, stretching before and after every workout is essential for beginning and experienced exercisers alike. Five to seven minutes in each case will do it.

There are also other pressing medical reasons to make a flexibility routine part of your warm-up and cool-down. It prepares your muscles for the exercise they are about to perform, but it also allows your heart to slowly accelerate to accommodate the work it's about to perform. As already mentioned, sudden, strenuous activity without proper warm-up can result in rapid and significant increases in both heart rate and blood pressure. Likewise, the cool-down stretching period gives your body time to readjust.

Flexibility exercises can also help build strength. When you're stretching one group of muscles, you inevitably contract other muscles to support your weight and hold the stretch. So in subtle ways your flexibility routine will also feed into your muscular strength building program. One final reason why flexing is such an important component of any overall fitness program relates to mind set. All of us, particularly executives, live under constant time pressure. If we're not careful, we treat our fitness program as just another hurdle in an already over-crowded day. A well-thought-out flexibility program gives you just enough time at the beginning and end of an exercise session to tune both your mind and body. It allows you to focus on the "here and now" of the exercise session. This is helpful for relaxing and focusing, and it's also a useful skill to carry out in the rest of your daily life.

Here's a good general routine you can perform before and after exercising. This routine should take you 3 to 4 minutes. In addition, you should warm up and cool down with 2 to 3 minutes of the activity you are using for exercise itself performed at a slow, relaxed pace. For example, if you are working out by swimming, warm up and cool down with 2 to 3 minutes of slow, relaxed swimming. During the warm-up phase, gradually increase the level of intensity and during the cool-down phase, gradually decrease the intensity.

1. *Neck stretches.* Lift your chin up slowly and tilt your head back; then bring your chin down to touch your chest. Repeat this process 3 to 4 times. Turn your head slowly to the right and glance over your right shoulder keeping the rest of your body still. Repeat in the opposite direction. Repeat this process 3 to 4 times.

2. *Shoulder shrugs.* Stand in a comfortable position with your feet shoulder-width apart. Lift your shoulders straight toward your head and relax. Repeat process 3 to 4 times.

3. *Side stretch.* Stand in a comfortable position with your feet shoulder-width apart. Extend your left arm over your head and bend your trunk directly to the right. Hold for 10 to 15 seconds. Repeat this process with the left arm bending the trunk directly to the right. Repeat 3 to 4 times on each side.

4. *Deltoid stretch.* Stand in a comfortable position. Grasp your left elbow with your right hand and gently pull your left arm across your body. Hold for 10 seconds. Switch arms and repeat the process in the other direction.

5. *Lower back stretch.* Lie flat on your back; bend your knees keeping your feet flat on the floor. Hug the left knee toward you as far as you can. Hold for 10 to 15 seconds. Repeat with the right leg.

6. *Lower leg stretch.* After the lower back stretch, remain with your back flat on the ground and bring both knees slowly to your chest. Hold for 10 to 15 seconds.

7. *Groin stretch.* Sit with your back straight and the soles of your feet together and as close to you as possible. Grasp your ankles and press downward with your elbows on your knees. Hold for 10 to 15 seconds. Repeat this process 2 to 3 times.

8. *Back and leg stretch.* Sit with your legs extended straight on either side of you as far as possible and your toes pointed upward. Lean out slowly between your legs until you feel a slight pull. Hold for 10 to 15 seconds.

9. *Calf stretch.* Stand with your right leg in front of you and bend the knee with the right foot flat on the ground. Keep the left leg straight behind you with the left foot flat on the ground. Lean forward over the right knee with your back straight. Hold for 10 to 15 seconds. Repeat with the other leg.

10. *Quadriceps stretch.* Use a chair for balance with this exercise. Stand on your right leg with your left arm holding the back of the chair. Bend your left leg backward at the knee and grasp your left foot with your right hand. Use your right hand to "cup" your foot between the ankle and toes. Pull the foot upward until you feel a slight pulling sensation in the front of the left thigh. Hold for 10 to 15 seconds. Repeat on the other side.

FIGURE 2. Yardstick and masking tape setup for flexibility testing.

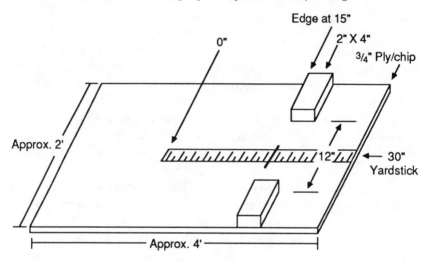

FIGURE 3. Procedure for testing yourself for flexibility.

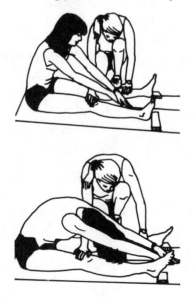

As you become an experienced exerciser, you will undoubtedly develop other stretches of your own. You might also ask an exercise specialist at your health club or corporate fitness facility to help you design a specific stretching routine geared to the activity you will be pursuing. In either case, know your limitations and level of flexibility before you jump into any program.

How can you test how "flexible" you are? One simple test, in use in many health clubs is called "sit and reach." To perform this test, it is important that you warm up properly using the stretching exercises already described. Then place a yardstick on the floor and put a piece of masking tape at the 15-inch mark (as shown in figure 2). Sit with the yardstick between your legs and with your heels about 10 to 12 inches apart and touching the edge of the masking tape, as shown in figure 3. Then slowly reach forward with both hands as far as possible and touch the yardstick, noting the inch marker you touch. Perform this maneuver three times. Avoid rapid, jerky motions which can cause muscle pulls. Your score is the farthest point on the yardstick you touched. Grade yourself according to the following standards.

	Inch Marker on Yardstick	Grade
Males	Greater than or equal to 21 inches	Excellent
	17–21 inches	Good
	13–17 inches	Average
	9–13 inches	Fair
	Less than 9 inches	Poor
Females	Greater than or equal to 23 inches	Excellent
	19–23 inches	Good
	15–19 inches	Average
	11–15 inches	Fair
	Less than 11 inches	Poor

More complex tests can be conducted at your health club or corporate fitness center. A physical therapist or athletic trainer can measure the flexibility of each joint, for example. Such measurements are particularly valuable where a preexisting injury to a joint or muscle has occurred and extra stretching and strengthening should be prescribed to prevent further injury.

4

Nutrition: Diets for a Lifetime

If I could turn back the clock ten years, knowing what I know now, I would have acted very differently. For one thing, I would have changed my diet. I was eating way too much in the way of fats—ice cream, peanut butter, and junk food, very high in sodium and extra calories and very low in good nourishment.

—K. W. REESE, executive vice-president
Tenneco, Inc.

The image of the corpulent executive is clearly a thing of the past. Proper nutrition and weight control have become top priorities in America's corporate suites. As one executive stated flatly: "The two-martini lunch is dead. The new power lunch is a salad and a piece of fruit."

The data from our survey of top executives corroborate this. More than 90% of the executives surveyed closely watch their diet, a concern that ranks a strong third behind regular exercise and not smoking as of "extreme importance" to them in maintaining their personal health. In particular, more than 60% try to avoid or minimize high-cholesterol foods and salt in their diets, while slightly more than half of the respondents try to limit high-fat dairy products, fried foods, sugar, and red meat. On the positive side, 82% of the executives pay attention to eating high-fiber foods—an average of more than seven times a week. Interestingly, of least concern is alcohol, which only 36% indicated they try to minimize or avoid.

Whatever healthy eating habits the executives try to maintain, it isn't easy much of the time. Many spoke of the unique dietary hurdles they

70

often face due to long working hours, frequent travel, and business meals. "My job requires a significant amount of travel. One of the real problems with that is it's so easy to gain weight having meals in nice restaurants around the country. I have at least three business meals a week and sometimes more," reported MCI's Don Steen in explaining one of the reasons why he's "always dieting." While most executives agree that eating on the road poses grave temptations, Federal-Mogul's chairman and CEO T. F. Russell takes advantage of the situation. "I find that I have less difficulty maintaining a balanced diet if I'm away from home for a week because I can order specifically what I want—the breakfast I want, or the lunch or dinner I want. Sometimes you're captive and you can't do that—you're served a steak or roast beef or something like that. But when I'm away, I can't walk past the refrigerator or bread box and grab things that I shouldn't grab."

Even when not traveling, frequent business meals pose a stiff challenge. "I have more damn breakfast meetings," lamented Robert Rowan, chairman and former CEO of Fruehauf. "I look at my schedule and sometimes in a six-day workweek, I'll have four breakfast meetings."

Incorporating proper diet into unpredictable schedules or long, irregular hours is a frequent problem, particularly for entrepreneurs. "I try to follow good nutritional patterns. I know the value of eating whole wheat, vegetables, and fruits. The problem is finding the time to have a balanced meal and not snacking," said one entrepreneur. "I've thought about having lunch brought in, catered by someone who makes nutritional meals. Now I have to find the time to find someone to do that!"

The temptation to substitute snacks or fast food for more nutritious meals grows in proportion to business pressures. Some of the entrepreneurs we interviewed recalled with some embarrassment their eating habits during the start-up phase of their companies. The experience of one *Inc.* CEO is distressingly common: "I would arrive at seven-thirty in the morning and often wouldn't leave until eight at night. Breakfast was coffee and doughnuts picked up on the way to the office. I always postponed lunch and then ended up skipping it. I'd have a cup of coffee. Then I'd realize, 'My God, it's eight P.M., I've got to go home.' On the way, I'd stop at the nearest pizza parlor and gorge myself. That was the pattern day after day. In the mornings, I'd be too tired to work out. I became fat. I felt heavy and sluggish, just like a machine where you neglect to change the oil."

You couldn't plan a diet worse for health and performance than the one described, even if you tried. For one, it's loaded with empty calories, caffeine, and cholesterol. Second, the timing of the calories is reversed. By mid-morning the executive's blood sugar would be low from the insulin response to the doughnuts so he would load up with caffeine from the coffee (probably liberally spiked with sugar just to add more empty calories). By the time he staggered from the office at the end of the day, he would load up on calories and fats, just prior to the time when his body least needed them—while he was sleeping.

If this entrepreneur's prior eating habits seem somewhat extreme, many other executives talk about their earlier years when they ate exactly what they wanted with little or no regard for the health consequences of their diet. "During my twenties, thirties, and early forties, there wasn't the knowledge that we have today about correct diets, particularly the impact of cholesterol and the whole cardiovascular issue," explained J. L. Ketelsen, Tenneco's chairman and CEO. "I ate a lot of what I consider bad food now. I didn't know any better."

Ketelsen's eating habits were "brought home dramatically to me by a bypass operation." "When I was recovering, somebody sent me a book on the Pritikin diet and exercise plan,* which I found very convincing, so my wife and I try to pattern our diet very closely to that." He used to eat "red meat and sweets," but Ketelsen now avoids all high-cholesterol foods and tries to stick "fundamentally to a lot of fish and fowl and broiled and stewed sorts of things, with little butter or fats of any kind."

Richard Snyder of Simon & Schuster is another executive who made major changes in his diet. "I grew up on chocolate cake and hot dogs and hamburgers. And I was taught it was all good for you, that stuff. Once I became knowledgeable about certain things to eat and not eat, I switched my diet," Snyder reported. "I have a chef who almost quits periodically because I won't let him cook the French way. Basically, I follow a very firm, proper diet. I eat veal, but no red meat, and I have fish three or four times a week. Occasionally, I'll have a sweet because I have a sweet tooth—I'll order dessert and have one spoonful."

Many executives have modified their diets after discovering specific health perils, such as high blood pressure or cholesterol levels. During a routine physical about 12 years ago, for example, Terry Jacobs of Jacor Communications discovered that his cholesterol level was too high. "My dad and uncle both died of heart-related problems before they hit

---

* The Pritikin plan, developed by Dr. Nathan Pritikin in the 1970s, emphasizes a low-fat, high-fiber diet as a means of fighting heart disease and cancer.

sixty," he noted. "So the exam scared me a bit. I was eating two eggs a day for breakfast, loved steaks and barbecued ribs—lots of things high in fat and cholesterol. I had to change. Although I don't totally abstain from red meat—I eat it maybe once a week—my diet is very heavy in chicken, fish, and veal. I seldom eat eggs or cheeses made with butter fat, and I don't eat regular butter or cream. I always drink skim milk."

If the health food knowledge revolution has altered the eating habits of top executives, it has also impacted menus in executive dining rooms. Fruit and cereal are common at executive breakfasts, and heavy sauces and desserts have virtually disappeared from dinner meeting fare. Restaurants have adapted to the nutritional trends, too. "In the last four or five years, everybody has become more health-conscious and, as a result, a lot more restaurants offer healthier foods. You go to a steak house today and you'll find fish on the menu, whereas five years ago that would be unheard of. At breakfast, they have more health cereals and fruits available. It's a lot easier to maintain a healthy diet, even if you have to eat out, than it used to be," observed Robert Rowan. "Still," he admitted, "I eat more when I'm on the road than when I'm at home. That's because my wife is also very health-conscious. She guards my diet with, I hate to admit it, greater diligence than I do."

Along with nutritional knowledge, the top executives have developed their own formulas for self-control. "I have a tendency to gain weight, and I watch it," explained one CEO, "and this is my strategy: I eliminate foods. I decided I wouldn't eat catsup or mayonnaise, so I just eliminated them from my diet. I've also eliminated soda, ice cream, things like that. I have pretty decent control. I like sweets, so sometimes it's a major decision. Should I have this cake or not? These cookies or these doughnuts, or not? When my resistance goes down, I stay out of the kitchen."

Although determined to maintain their nutritional regimens, the executives do admit that there are occasional lapses and weaknesses. "I have a diet from a dietitian and I try to stick with the guidelines. I might have an apple up until eight or nine o'clock at night, but not after that. Sometimes, though, I cheat like hell on weekends. I'll really indulge in popcorn and pretzels and things like that," said one. After describing his strict dietary program, another admitted: "Now, I'm also the kind of guy who will go out once in a while and have a big ice cream sundae or a pizza."

As with other facets of their personal and professional lives, most of the executives try to maintain a balanced outlook when it comes to nutrition and simply incorporate their programs into their life-styles without letting them become a total preoccupation. As Ronald Thomas, chairman and former president of Ciprico, Inc., observed: "I'm very conscious of my eating habits and, compared to the average person, I think I do a pretty good job of avoiding a lot of foods. But I'm not paranoid about it. I'll eat a hamburger or steak or something like that once in a while. Generally, though, if I have a choice between chicken and beef, I pick the chicken."

Executives watch their nutrition carefully for two basic reasons: They want to feel good and they want to look good. The health hazards of poor nutrition have been well publicized; they know that the risk of heart disease, stroke, diabetes, certain cancers, and obesity can be affected by their diet. "I eat well because I don't want to have a heart attack," said one CEO, matter-of-factly. They also know that what they eat can affect their energy level and ability to perform. Many reported feeling "sluggish" and "irritable" when they don't eat properly.

Top executives also care very strongly about how they look. Simple vanity is one reason. Another is that there is a strong prejudice against overweight executives. Not a single executive we interviewed was significantly overweight. Time and time again, they referred to their management teams as "lean and aggressive" and admitted that carrying extra pounds can work against the careers of executives on the rise. "Part of an executive's responsibility is to represent the company and part of that is personal appearance," explained Kenneth Otto, senior vice-president at Tenneco. "When we think about promotions, it may come up. How does he look? How does he represent Tenneco?"

The CEO of an entrepreneurial firm put it more bluntly: "When I'm interviewing people, I want to know what they do for health and fitness, and I ask. I made the mistake of hiring a fat person once. He had a very low energy level and just couldn't keep up the pace. We need to look fit and act fit. Maybe ten or even twenty pounds is OK, but anything more than that is really not acceptable."

While there is strong interest in nutrition among top executives, there are also major gaps in specific knowledge and practices. For example, 64% of the executives surveyed did not know their cholesterol level, a shockingly high percentage considering the risk of heart disease posed by high cholesterol. In my clinical experience, other knowledge gaps among executives are often as distressing. Part of the problem is that they are functioning on out-of-date data or insufficient information on nutrition and weight control. It comes as a shock to some that certain foods that they had thought for years were good for them are actually very unhealthy. Others are appalled by the fact that the diets they had been following so religiously may actually be doing more harm than good. Still others have no conception about the different types of fats they consume and the fatty foods that are the worst for them.

In nutrition, perhaps more than in any other health-related field, knowledge is power. During the past five years, scientific and medical research has added important new findings to our understanding of diet and weight control. To examine some of the issues that concern executives and to clear up common misconceptions, let's look at eight specific diet factors: cholesterol, fats, fiber, salt, sugar, caffeine, alcohol, and vitamins.

CHOLESTEROL

One would have to have been comatose for the past five years to not have learned something about cholesterol and its relation to heart disease. Yet it is clear that both the public and the medical community have a long way to go. A recent survey by the National Institutes of Health (NIH) showed that only 30% of physicians regard controlling cholesterol levels to be as important as controlling hypertension and avoiding cigarettes in the prevention of coronary heart disease (CHD). As a cardiologist, I find this particularly alarming because it leads to a significant amount of undertreatment of elevated cholesterol levels, leaving millions of people at higher risk than they should be for heart disease.

The average American consumes 400 to 500 milligrams of cholesterol a day—almost 50% higher than the amount recommended by the American Heart Association (AHA). It's not surprising, then, that more than 50% of American adults have blood cholesterol levels exceeding 200 milligrams per deciliter (mg/dl), dangerously above the 130 to 190 mg/dl guideline recommended by the 1987 *National Cholesterol Education Program Expert Panel Report.*

From our survey, it is clear that portions of the message of lowering cholesterol have gotten through to the highest levels of corporate America. More than 63% of our respondents try to minimize high-cholesterol foods in their diets. Yet only 33% actually knew their cholesterol levels. Furthermore, only 51% attempt to minimize red meat in their diets, apparently unaware that red meat is a major source of cholesterol in the American diet. Many executives don't realize that egg yolks are the largest single source of cholesterol in the American diet.

It seems somewhat paradoxical that so many executives know they should try to reduce cholesterol, yet so few know their own level or understand specifically how to reduce it. Yet, these findings are consistent with my experience in teaching executives about cholesterol.

Several years ago, for example, I spoke to 600 top executives from a high-technology firm at their annual sales conference. Prior to the conference I asked them to fill out a questionnaire about their health attitudes. More than 90% said they attempted to avoid high-cholesterol foods in their daily diet. After sharing this striking bit of information with them, I asked how many had eaten eggs for breakfast that morning. More than half of those in the audience raised their hands. Then I asked how many had eaten more than two eggs that morning. Still more than half the audience had their hands raised. Those who raised their hands to the second question had already eaten twice the average amount of daily dietary cholesterol recommended by the AHA—and lunch and dinner were yet to come.

OK, you say, but you've already cut way back on the number of eggs in your diet, so that doesn't apply to you. Unfortunately, it's not that simple. Cholesterol can appear in a lot of places where you don't suspect it. Red meat and eggs are major culprits, but so are milk, cheese, and butter— common ingredients in many baked foods and sauces (see table on page 78). In addition, many of these cholesterol culprits contain saturated fats, which make the problem worse since they impair cholesterol processing, often resulting in elevated blood cholesterol levels.

What exactly is cholesterol? Cholesterol is a naturally occurring waxy substance found only in animal tissues, particularly eggs, dairy products, meat, poultry, fish, and shellfish. It is not found in plants. It makes up an important part of the membranes of the cell wall structure in the human body and plays a role in the production of a number of hormones, including the sex hormones. A certain amount of cholesterol is therefore essential to life. It is only when too much cholesterol is present in the bloodstream that it causes problems. Fatty deposits that contain cholesterol collect in the inner walls of blood vessels and arteries, and contribute to a condition called atherosclerosis, or progressive narrowing of the arteries with fatty plaque. This buildup impedes the flow of blood to the heart and, when severe enough, can cause a heart attack.

Recently, there has been a lot of attention to several "subfractions" of cholesterol—namely HDL (high-density lipoprotein) cholesterol and LDL (low-density lipoprotein) cholesterol. The names are derived from the type of carrier molecules, or lipoproteins, that transport cholesterol through the bloodstream to cells throughout the body. LDL is the major cholesterol carrier in the blood. High levels of LDL have been linked to coronary artery disease, earning it the reputation as the "bad" cholesterol. HDL has been associated with a reduction in the likelihood of developing coronary disease (by helping transport "bad" cholesterol out of the bloodstream), and thus has been labeled "good" cholesterol. Research shows that LDL cholesterol levels can be reduced by carefully monitoring the types of fats in your diet. Regular aerobic exercise can increase your HDL cholesterol.

What does all this mean to the average executive? First, every executive should know his or her cholesterol level and if it is elevated, should be doing something definite about it. There is no longer any question that elevated blood cholesterol is a major risk factor for coronary heart disease. Tight control of cholesterol, therefore, is an essential health precaution. There is a prevalent "it will never happen to me" attitude among self-confident, ostensibly healthy executives. Just because you seem to be feeling great, however, doesn't necessarily mean your arteries are.

Determining your cholesterol level involves a simple blood test that can be easily incorporated into periodic visits to your physician. If the initial reading is elevated, a second "fasting" sample (drawn before you have breakfast in the morning, with no food after midnight the night before) should be taken to allow determination of HDL and LDL levels. I recommend that this cholesterol level be measured at least once every two years in individuals over age 30 and more often if the cholesterol level is elevated.

Second, executives should be more aggressive in pushing "average" cholesterol levels lower. Among the 33% who knew their cholesterol level, the average was 220 mg/dl. While this is consistent with the average for the American population, in their age group, it is too high. According to both the AHA and the NIH, the ideal range for adults in our society is 130 to 190 mg/dl.

To many people, including physicians, these guidelines may seem overly restrictive. However, let's put the 220 mg/dl of our executives in perspective. We now know that the risk of developing CHD begins to accelerate rapidly above the level of 200 mg/dl. If an individual has a

CHOLESTEROL CONTENT OF FOODS

Food Item	Serving	Cholesterol (mg)
Meats, Poultry, and Fish		
BEEF		
Frankfurter	2, cooked	61
Sausage, cured	2, cooked	67
Rib eye, lean, broiled	3½ oz., cooked	80
Top round, lean, broiled	3½ oz., cooked	84
Liver, braised	3½ oz., cooked	389
Kidneys, simmered	3½ oz., cooked	387
LAMB		
Leg, lean, roasted	3½ oz., cooked	89
Loin chop, broiled	3½ oz., cooked	94
PORK		
Loin, lean, roasted	3½ oz., cooked	93
Liverwurst	3½ oz.	158
VEAL		
Cutlet, medium fat, braised	3½ oz., cooked	128
POULTRY		
Chicken, stewed, light meat, w/o skin	3½ oz., cooked	70
Turkey, roasted	3½ oz., cooked	86
Turkey frankfurter	2	101
FISH		
Tuna, canned, in oil	2 oz.	37
Perch, dry heat	3½ oz., cooked	42
Lobster, northern	3½ oz., cooked	72
Haddock, dry heat	3½ oz., cooked	74
Crab, blue, moist heat	3½ oz., cooked	100
Shrimp, moist heat	3½ oz., cooked	195
Dairy and Egg Products		
MILK		
Yogurt, plain, low fat	4 oz.	2
Skim milk	8 oz.	4
Yogurt, plain, regular fat	4 oz.	14
Whole milk	8 oz.	33

CHOLESTEROL CONTENT OF FOODS

Food Item	Serving	Cholesterol (mg)
CHEESE		
Cottage cheese, low fat	4 oz.	5
Mozzarella, part skim	1 oz.	16
Feta	1 oz.	25
American, processed	1 oz.	27
Brie	1 oz.	28
Cheddar	1 oz.	30
Cream cheese	1 oz.	31
EGGS		
Egg, chicken, white	1	0
Egg, chicken, yolk	1	272
Egg, chicken, whole	1	274
Frozen Desserts		
Pudding pops	1 pop	1
Sherbet, orange	1 cup	14
Ice milk, soft serve	1 cup	18
Ice cream, vanilla, 16% fat	1 cup	88
Ice cream, French vanilla, soft serve	1 cup	153
Other Foods		
Bagel	1	0
Cornflakes, w/o milk	1 cup	0
Lima beans	1 cup, cooked	0
Pita bread	½ large	0
Rice, white	1 cup, cooked	0
Spaghetti, cooked	1 cup	0
Mayonnaise	1 tablespoon	8
Chocolate chip cookies	4	18
Plain doughnut	1	20
Corn chips	1 oz.	25
Fig bars	4	27
Sour cream sauce	½ cup	45
Egg noodles	1 cup, cooked	50
Pizza, cheese	⅛ of 15″ pizza	56
Pound cake	1/17 of loaf	64
Béarnaise sauce	½ cup	99
Waffle, 7″ diameter	1	102
Lemon meringue pie	⅙ of 9″ pie	143
Quiche lorraine	⅛ of 8″ quiche	285

Source: Reprinted from "Eating to Lower Your High Blood Cholesterol," National Institutes of Health Publication No. 87-2920, 1987. Originally published by the National Heart, Lung, and Blood Institute.

cholesterol level of 200 mg/dl, his chance of developing CHD is *half* that of an individual with a level of 250 mg/dl. Put another way, the person with the lower cholesterol level can reasonably expect to delay the onset of significant atherosclerosis, if it develops to that extent at all, by 10 years compared with his counterpart with the higher level.

If the bad news is that the average cholesterol level among executives is too high, the good news is that the technique to lower these levels is simple, painless, and well within your reach. Simply by making a conscious effort to minimize cholesterol and saturated fat intake, the average individual can lower his or her cholesterol level by 10% to 15%. For the respondents to our survey, this would drop cholesterol levels below 200 mg/dl, close to the range recommended by the AHA. Recent NIH studies demonstrated that aggressive treatment of elevated cholesterol can significantly reduce the likelihood of heart disease, and one study even showed regression of established CHD in individuals whose cholesterol was tightly controlled.

In its dietary guidelines, the AHA recommends that cholesterol intake should be less than 100 milligrams per 1,000 calories and should not exceed 300 milligrams a day. I typically advise executives who have neither the time nor the inclination to keep an exact running tally of their cholesterol intake to pay much closer attention to what they eat (beware the "hidden" cholesterol in the ingredients of many foods) and adopt a "prudent" style of eating. By this I mean eating no more than two eggs a week, no more than two servings of red meat per week, drinking low-fat milk, and avoiding other high-cholesterol/high-fat foods.

Two other cholesterol-related topics deserve mention: weight and exercise. First, there are many reasons to maintain an ideal body weight, and cholesterol is one of them. There is a strong relation between obesity and elevated cholesterol levels. One of the first measures I stress with overweight executives who have elevated cholesterol levels is that they lose weight and keep it off. Second, regular aerobic exercise has been clearly linked to raising the HDL ("good") fraction of the proteins that carry cholesterol. Exercise can help reduce the likelihood of developing CHD if you also watch your diet and don't overcompensate for your activity with high-cholesterol foods.

FATS

There are many reasons to reduce the amount of fat in your diet. A high dietary intake of fats has been linked to heart disease, diabetes, and increased incidence of colon cancer. Further, fats are a major contributor to obesity. Ounce for ounce, fat has more than *twice* the calories of carbohydrates or proteins. Our survey suggests that this message has begun to get through to executives—more than 53% make an effort to limit high-fat dairy products and fried foods in their diet.

There are basically three types of fats: saturated, monounsaturated, and polyunsaturated. Animal fats tend to be saturated and are usually solid at room temperature, whereas plant and vegetable fats tend to be monounsaturated or polyunsaturated and are generally liquid at room temperature. There are exceptions, of course. For example, coconut oil, palm oil, and chocolate are all high in saturated fats.

Saturated fats tend to raise blood cholesterol. Both monounsaturated and polyunsaturated fats may reduce cholesterol. The monounsaturated fats may be the best choice of all since they selectively lower LDL (the worst type of cholesterol), whereas polyunsaturated fats have been shown in some studies to lower both LDL and HDL. Examples of monounsaturated fats include olive oil, peanut oil, and stick margarine. Polyunsaturated fats include safflower oil, sunflower oil, corn oil, and sesame oil.

Saturated Fats		Monounsaturated Fats		Polyunsaturated Fats	
Animal Sources	**Plant Sources**	**Animal Sources**	**Plant Sources**	**Animal Sources (of omega-3 fatty acids)**	**Plant Sources**
Cheese	Coconut oil	Chicken	Vegetable shortening	Fish	Almonds
Butter	Palm oil	Fish	Avocados		Walnuts
Milk	Palm kernel oil		Pecans		Filberts
Meat	Cocoa butter		Olive oil		Soft margarine
Eggs	(chocolate)		Canola oil		Sesame oil
Lard			Stick margarine		Mayonnaise
Pork			Peanut oil		Soybean oil
			Peanut butter		Corn oil
			Cottonseed oil		Sunflower oil
					Safflower oil

Source: Compiled by the author.

While this may sound complex, the bottom line is simple: There are many important health reasons to reduce the amount of fat in your diet, particularly animal fats. The AHA guidelines suggest a total fat intake of less than 30% of total calories (approximately 15% protein and 55% carbohydrates). Saturated fat intake should be less than 10% of calories, and, ideally, only 10% of total fat consumed. Realistically, only a committed health fanatic might be expected to keep track of these percentages. But you should be alert to the volume and types of fats you consume. Easy techniques for reducing animal fats, for example, include trimming fat from meats (preferably before cooking), avoiding processed foods, and substituting low-fat dairy products for higher fat varieties.

FIBER

Most executives recognize the importance of eating adequate fiber. More than 82% of our survey respondents make it a point to include high-fiber foods in their diets. High-fiber cereals might well be called "The Breakfast of Executives." Few go to the lengths of John Bierwirth, who eats homemade granola for breakfast, but all of the executives we interviewed have made a conscious effort to eat more whole grains, fruits, and cereals. Noted Xerox's Paul Allaire: "I eat much less red meat now than five years ago, and I'm much more concerned about fiber— those are the major dietary concessions I've made."

The emphasis on fiber grew out of the 1970s and is largely attributed to Dr. Dennis Burkitt, an esteemed English physician, who observed that cultures where more fiber was ingested than in Western cultures had a lower incidence of cancers of the colon and rectum. Burkitt's findings, although widely debated in the scientific literature, spawned a number of popular books and articles. Almost overnight, fiber consumption in the United States skyrocketed.

Fiber comes from the cell walls and other components of plants. It cannot be broken down by enzymes in the human digestive system and thus passes through the system and is eliminated in the stool. There are two basic types of fiber: water soluble and insoluble. Insoluble fiber absorbs water in the gastrointestinal tract, making stools softer and bulkier, which facilitates elimination. It helps reduce intestinal problems such as constipation, hemorrhoids, and diverticulosis. Insoluble fiber has also been linked to a reduction in the risk of developing colon cancer, although this is debated in the medical community and much more research remains to be done. Good sources of insoluble fiber are wheat and bran, the outer husks of whole grains, and certain vegetables like broccoli, cabbage, and peppers. Some fruits such as apples, pears, and strawberries also provide insoluble fiber.

Soluble fibers, which also help your internal plumbing stay in regular working order, have been associated with a reduction in cholesterol levels, thus lowering the risk of heart disease. Good sources of soluble fiber are oatmeal, legumes (peas, and the like), fruit, and certain vegetables (see table on page 84).

In addition to aiding your digestive system and lowering the risk of cancer and high cholesterol, there's another excellent reason why high-fiber foods are important: Foods high in fiber tend to be low in fat and calories. Thus they play a role in weight management.

Busy executives who opt for fast-food meals commonly have a low fiber intake. Who has time to munch on an apple? Much less peel an orange? Or sit down to a bowl of oatmeal when you can grab a dough-nut? There are any number of non-time-consuming ways you can incor-porate fruits, vegetables, and whole grains into your diet. Instead of a doughnut, have a bran, blueberry, or corn muffin. Instead of saltines or cheese crackers, have wheat, rye, or rice crackers. Instead of potato chips, substitute an apple or popcorn (unbuttered and unsalted, of course).

For executives who want to know more precisely how much fiber they should be consuming, I recommend at least 25 grams a day. There are many choices within the two basic fiber groups (insoluble and soluble), and I generally advise eating a variety of both. For some executives, however, moderation may be the watchword. If you already have bowel problems (such as hemorrhoids or diverticular disease), don't dramati-cally increase your fiber intake on your own. Consult your physician first.

For most adults, the advice of *New York Times* health columnist Jane Brody makes sense—add a salad a day to the old prescription of an apple a day to keep the doctor away.

SALT

There is far too much salt in the average American's diet. The typical adult in our society consumes between 6 and 8 grams of salt a day—a

FIBER SCOREBOARD

Food	Amount	Fiber (g)
Fresh fruit (raw or cooked, w/skin)		
Apples, pears, berries	1 piece for ½ cup	4.0
All others	1 piece for ½ cup	1.5
Canned fruit (w/o skin)	½ cup	1.5
Dried fruit	½ cup	4.0
Fresh vegetables (raw or cooked)		
Peas, parsnips	½ cup	5.0
Potatoes	1 baked w/skin	4.0
Corn, squash, tomatoes	½ cup	2.0
Cabbage family, carrots	½ cup	2.0
All others	½ cup	1.5
Tossed salad greens	1 cup	1.5
Cereal: cooked whole grain	½ cup	2.5
Bran types	½ cup	4.0
Granola, whole grain	½ cup	2.5
Refined	½ cup	1.0
Bread: whole grain	1 slice	2.5
Refined	1 slice	1.0
Bran muffin	1 muffin	3.0
Crackers: whole grain	3 rye wafers/6 small	2.5
Graham crackers	2 squares	1.5
Refined	6 small	.5
Popcorn	1 cup	3.0
Pasta, rice: whole grain	1 cup, cooked	3.0
Refined	1 cup, cooked	1.0
Nuts, seeds	¼ cup, 2 oz.	5.0
Legumes	½ cup	6.0
Meat, cheese, fats, most sweets		0

Source: Kapitan, R.: The Newtrition Workshop.

frighteningly high figure compared with the maximum 3 grams per day recommended by the AHA. One of the problems is that infants and young people consume far too much salt and it becomes an acquired taste. Many adults, having become used to the taste of overly salted foods as they grew up, regard it as normal or even desirable. Sodium reduction appears to have made headway among executives, however. More than 63% of those who responded to our survey reported that they try to minimize the amount of salt they eat.

There is now some evidence, although still hotly debated, that overexposure to salt contributes to the development of high blood pressure. Certainly, if you have high blood pressure or a family history of it, you should dramatically reduce your salt intake. Even if you don't, you should limit the amount of salt in your diet as a basic health precaution.

Some of the steps for doing this are very simple. Never reach for the saltshaker before tasting your food. A lot of meals are too highly salted even before they reach the table. President Ronald Reagan cited "eliminating the saltshaker" from his table as one of the prescriptions for his long and vigorous life. It's good advice, and not as hard as you might imagine to follow. At least if you have to get up from the table to get the shaker, you may give it a second thought.

You can substantially lower salt intake by substituting natural foods, such as fruits and vegetables, for processed snack foods. And, finally, read food labels! Salt appears in unsuspected places, and food does not have to taste "salty" to contain large quantities of sodium. Some breakfast cereals, for example, are loaded with sodium, as are a number of condiments, soups, cheeses, baked goods, and packaged cookies.

SUGAR

Most of the sugar eaten in the United States is refined (purified) sugar contained in processed foods. Candy, canned fruits, jellies, and soft drinks all contain large amounts of sugar, as do ice cream and many bakery products. As a source of energy, our bodies use natural sugars— such as those found in fruits—and refined sugars in the same way. However, when sugar is refined, the process also removes vitamins and other nutrients. Fruits supply valuable vitamins and minerals; refined sugars do not. They are simply a source of "energy" calories with no other nutritional value.

By any criteria, Americans consume an enormous amount of sugar. The average person consumes almost a quarter of his or her daily calories as sugar, and more than half of this is refined. This amounts to 600 calories a day, or an incredible 128 pounds of sugar a year consumed by the average American.

Most executives don't pay enough attention to sugars in their diets.

Only about 50% of our survey respondents consciously try to avoid or minimize refined sugars and sweets. It may be that many simply don't have a sweet tooth. Based on our interviews, however, it would appear to be just the opposite. Cutting down on sugar calories is an ongoing struggle for most executives. Some are obviously more aware than others of just what that daily indulgence (deserved after a hard day at the office) can do to their health in the long run.

The major health problem linked to sugar consumption is tooth decay. It has long been recognized that candy and sweets can damage the teeth; they can also be harmful to the gums. Sugars on the teeth or at the gum line are avidly consumed by bacteria in the mouth, which generate waste products harmful to both teeth and gums. The problem is not the consumption of sugars per se, but eating sweets at or between meals in forms that are likely to stick to the teeth and remain in the mouth. Among the biggest culprits are raisins and other dried fruits, marshmallow crème, and caramel. Also, as we get older, sugar can increase the potential for periodontal problems.

Another problem with foods high in sugar is that they contain a huge amount of calories in proportion to the bulk or hunger satisfaction they provide. A candy bar or slice of apple pie with ice cream, for example, will give you a huge number of calories (more than 25 percent of what you need for the day) but may not give you the sensation of "being full." Although there is no direct evidence that a high-sugar intake is linked with obesity, it's intuitively obvious that the two often go hand-in-hand. Why? Because many foods packed with sugar are also sources of fat— cakes, pies, cookies, ice cream, candy bars, and other sweet treats. It's almost a given that when fats are cut out of the diet, sugar intake is reduced.

A particularly troublesome myth for the executive is the idea that a candy bar in the middle of the afternoon will serve as a needed "pick-me-up." Unfortunately, just the opposite is likely. A sugar-laden candy bar will cause your blood sugar to rise transiently and stimulate the pancreas to secrete insulin, thus resulting in a rapid return of the blood sugar to the initial level, or even lower. A piece of fruit is a much better solution if you're taking a break.

One noteworthy villain in the sugar story is soft drinks. A 12-ounce can of soft drink may contain up to nine teaspoons of sugar and 150 to 180 calories. The average executive in our survey drinks 10 cans of soft drinks a week. (At an average of 520 cans a year, this is still below the national average for adults—more than 600 cans a year!) The encouraging news is that two-thirds of our sample drink *diet* soft drinks.

As everyone knows, the diet soft drink market has mushroomed in the past few years, thanks to the development of low-calorie sweeteners such as NutraSweet™ (aspartame) and saccharin. And, of course, these sweeteners aren't limited to soft drinks. Literally hundreds of food products—from cereals and cocoa mixes to desserts, salad dressings, and tea—are sweetened with either NutraSweet™ or saccharin. Many consumers regularly use these reduced-calorie products in place of the traditional products. Is there an advantage to doing this? Most definitely! A quick glance at the table below shows that calories can be saved by using low-calorie sweeteners.

Product	Calories with Sugar*	Calories with Low-cal Sweeteners*	Calories Saved
Soft drink (12 oz.)	150	1	149
Gelatin dessert (½ cup)	81	10	71
Dry mix lemonade (8 oz.)	86	5	81
Coffee (1 cup)	35	4	31
Chocolate pudding (½ cup)	177	75	102

Source: Calorie Control Council Commentary, Vol. 10, No. 1, 1988.
*Estimate.

Of course, it does no good to use these reduced-calorie products if the calories saved are consumed by eating high-calorie foods. The trick is to enjoy these low-calorie foods and watch your fat and sugar intake over the course of the day.

Sugar is an important source of energy and should not be eliminated from your diet. However, if weight is a problem, be particularly careful about those calorie-packed pick-me-ups that don't work and are detrimental to the battle of the bulge. The natural sugars in fruits are an effective substitute for the empty calories of candy, cakes, and sodas.

CAFFEINE

People who say that they can't really function in the morning before their first cup of coffee may be partially correct—the caffeine in their coffee is a mild stimulant that affects many of the body's organs, including the brain and central nervous system, heart, and gastrointestinal tract. It may be a needed stimulant, but it also can cause jitters (so-called coffee nerves), palpitations, headaches, and insomnia. And, it's addictive.

While coffee is the major source of caffeine, it is also found in tea, cola drinks, and, in smaller amounts, in chocolate. The average American drinks 450 cups of coffee a year—or just over 8 cups a week. That's nothing compared with the respondents to our survey, who consume an average of 20 cups a week or a staggering 1,040 cups a year. Only about one-third of those indicated that they drink decaffeinated coffee, making top executives the true addicts among the nation's coffee lovers.

Overall, only 40% of the executives surveyed attempt to minimize caffeine-containing beverages in their daily diet. Is this so bad? Is caffeine really a health hazard? Medical research on this point is inconclusive. A couple of studies have suggested that elevated cholesterol levels and heart disease are more common in individuals who consume large amounts of caffeine. These studies have been disputed, and nobody has drawn a causal link between caffeine and CHD. Excessive consumption of caffeine has also occasionally been linked to increased incidence of cancer (particularly bladder cancer), but the data are unconvincing.

The best advice is to drink coffee in moderation and pay attention to how you personally respond to it. Difficulty in sleeping, jitters, palpitations, or headaches all signal reasons to cut down on coffee or other caffeine-containing beverages.

ALCOHOL

Alcohol poses a variety of health risks. Excessive consumption of it is associated with a two- to threefold increase in cancer of the larynx, esophagus, and liver. When combined with cigarette smoking, the incidence of laryngeal and esophageal cancers skyrocket to more than 10 times the average.

Yet, used in moderation, alcohol poses minimal risk and may even provide some positive health benefits. What's "moderate" consumption? Most studies define it as no more than two 12-ounce glasses of beer, two 5-ounce glasses of wine, or one 1½-ounce "shot" of distilled spirits a day. Several studies have suggested that individuals who consume moderate amounts of alcohol live longer than either teetotalers or excessive drinkers. In one study of Hawaiian males, those who drank two beers a day had less heart disease than those who completely abstained.

Executive attitudes toward alcohol have changed dramatically in the past 10 years or so. Moderation is in, excessive drinking is out. Alcohol at lunch is shunned, if not frowned upon. Tenneco's J. L. Ketelsen summarized the prevailing mood: "People understand more about physical wellness. They recognize that if you have two martinis at lunch and go back to your desk, you're far more likely to fall asleep than to be productive. Life-styles have changed. Most people can't stand the calories from alcohol because the waistline starts to show it—giving them more than one reason to cut it out." This CEO is right on target. Gram for gram, alcohol provides almost as many calories as fat, seven calories per gram of alcohol compared with nine calories per gram of fat. And alcohol calories are definitely empty calories. That's basically all you get from a can of beer or a glass of wine . . . calories.

Only 36% of the executives in our survey were trying to minimize

Caloric Content of Some Common Alcoholic Beverages

Beverage	Serving Size	Calories
Beer (4.5% alcohol by volume)	12 fl. oz.	151
Gin, rum, vodka, whiskey		
80-proof	1 jigger	97
86-proof	1 jigger	105
90-proof	1 jigger	110
96-proof	1 jigger	116
100-proof	1 jigger	124
Wines		
Dessert (18.8% alcohol by volume)		
Wineglass	1 glass	141
Sherryglass	1 glass	81
Table (12.2% alcohol by volume)		
Wineglass	1 glass	87

Source: United States Department of Agriculture, Nutritive Value of American Foods in Common Units, Handbook 456, 1975.

their alcohol consumption, a statistic explained by the fact that most of them do not drink that much to begin with. Among the respondents, the average executive drinks beer, wine, or hard liquor three to four times a week, and the average amount consumed each time is less than two drinks. Almost one-third never drink, rarely drink, or drink less than once a week.

Besides the two-martini lunches, the days of corporate bashes are numbered. Excessive drinking, particularly at company functions, is no longer regarded as a healthy way of letting off steam. "Twenty years ago, with some frequency, company parties turned into real drunks. It was quite acceptable to laugh and reminisce about it the next day," observed Navistar's Donald Lennox. "You just don't see that anymore. It's much less accepted and taken as a sign of lack of self-discipline, even immaturity."

VITAMINS

Busy executives often ask me for advice about vitamins. After all, the story typically goes, "I'm too busy to eat a balanced diet and a daily vitamin tablet can't hurt." I can agree with at least part of the statement—one daily multivitamin pill probably won't hurt you, but, by the same token, it almost certainly won't help you.

Our species survived for millennia without the aid of specially designated vitamin capsules. The fact remains: Sound, balanced nutrition is the best and easiest way to be sure you get all the essential vitamins, minerals, and other substances you need. Taking vitamins on top of your normal diet is a good way to increase the vitamin content of your urine.

There are a few exceptions to this general statement. If you are a heavy drinker (by "heavy" I mean four or more shots of liquor or highballs a day), you should take a daily multivitamin. That's because your alcohol intake interferes with the normal absorption of vitamins: You're probably not eating an adequate diet, and the vitamins are needed to help repair the chronic damage done to your body by alcohol. Some people with gastrointestinal diseases also need vitamin supplements because of abnormal absorption in the stomach and intestines.

The bottom line for the average adult, however, is that vitamins are a waste of money. That includes vitamin C, by the way, despite some fairly extravagant claims for it as a cold fighter. In contrast to supplementation with a daily multivitamin, which is a waste but relatively harmless, megadoses of vitamins can actually be dangerous, and I know of no demonstrated medical benefits (with the possible exception of taking niacin for elevated blood cholesterol).

One final, related area: In recent years, there has been an increasing number of "total eating systems," which typically contain some vitamin pills, fiber bars (or the equivalent), fish-oil pills, and the like. The only proven benefit of these regimens is to the companies that manufacture them. Avoid them.

WEIGHT CONTROL

By far the most prevalent nutritional concern among executives in our study was maintaining proper weight. Many spoke of weight control as a "constant battle" that required daily vigilance; even those who appeared slim referred to periods of inactivity and overindulgence when they had put on weight.

If obesity presents an image problem for an executive, it also poses significant health risks. Obesity is associated with high blood pressure, diabetes, elevated cholesterol, and risk of certain cancers and puts additional strain on every organ system—particularly the heart, bones, and joints. In fact, obesity is a major health problem. Using the very liberal criterion of allowing a person to be 20% over ideal weight before regarding it as a serious health risk, more than 8 million adult males and 16 million adult females in our society carry this serious risk factor. A 50-year-old who is carrying 25% extra weight cuts his life expectancy by a decade.

The diet industry in the United States is a multibillion-dollar enterprise. Next year there will be at least one diet book on the *New York Times* best-seller list, as there has been for the past 20 years. The reason for this is quite simple: Virtually none of the diets works in the long term. Almost any reasonable diet where calories are restricted will work in the short run; however, without fundamental changes in the way a person eats and exercises, weight is almost invariably regained. Carefully controlled scientific studies have shown that of people who lose weight by dieting, more than 95% will have gained it back within one to two years. The people who dieted last year will typically have gained back most of the weight by this year and thus be ready to purchase the next "miracle" diet that comes along.

91

It used to be thought that obesity was primarily caused by overeating. Now we know that inactivity plays as big a role. Obese people typically eat less than lean people. At the same time, they are much less active. The principles of weight management and weight loss are deceptively simple. To lose weight, you must expend more calories than you take in. In other words, you must find a way to tip the energy balance in your favor. There are three ways to do this: dieting (you decrease the number of calories you take in); exercise (you increase the number of calories you expend); or a combination of dieting and exercise. Study after study have shown that the combination of dieting and exercise is most effective for weight loss.

When you attempt to lose weight by restricting your calories alone (dieting), about two-thirds of the weight you lose is fat and about one-third muscle. When you gain that weight back, almost all of it will be gained back as fat. Thus, you are actually in a less favorable position than when you started because your percentage of body fat has increased. This is the central problem in the "yo-yo" dieting syndrome that all too many adults become trapped in.

The major reason why it's so hard to lose weight by dieting alone is that the body has a series of defenses that come into play to defend whatever weight you're at. (Some people have called this "set point.") When you try to lose weight by cutting back on calories, your body will resist you in at least two important ways. First, your brain will send signals that you are hungry: You'll find yourself spending a lot of time thinking about food. Second, your basal metabolic rate (BMR), which measures the number of calories you expend going about your daily activities, will slow down. When you reduce the number of calories you take in, your body interprets that as a "semistarvation" mode and starts slowing down systems to preserve current weight.

There are a number of reasons why adding exercise to the weight-management equation works so well. First, exercise counteracts the tendency of the BMR to decrease when the number of calories consumed is reduced. When you add an exercise component to your weight-management regimen, the BMR remains approximately what it was before you started dieting.

Second, regular aerobic exercise helps maintain lean muscle while fat is lost. Most people who are overweight are actually "overfat." What they need to do is selectively lose fat. Exercise ensures that muscle is preserved and that weight loss is indeed fat loss. In one study of overweight men, for example, subjects were asked to walk for 90 minutes a day for eight weeks. At the end of the study, the average weight loss was 15 pounds. Most importantly, lean muscle mass had been preserved and almost all of the weight lost was fat. Thus, exercise is the best way to combat the danger of yo-yo dieting.

Finally, exercise is a good way to burn extra calories. To lose a pound of fat you must burn an extra 3,500 calories. When people look at exercise charts and see how many miles they need to walk or run or swim in order to do this, they often get inappropriately discouraged. What they fail to realize is that relatively modest amounts of exercise performed consistently can result in very significant weight loss. For example, executives are often surprised when I tell them that if they go out for a brisk walk for 45 minutes four times a week *and* don't increase the amount they eat, they will lose 18 pounds over the course of a year. More important, virtually all of this weight loss will be fat loss, which is what the overweight person needs to accomplish.

From our survey, it appears that the exercise component of weight control is commonly ascribed to by top executives. When asked why they exercise, 65% listed weight control as one of the major reasons. Still, as they attested, it takes a sense of determination—even a sense of mission—to keep the scales in balance. For some who had earlier weight problems, it even meant a somewhat dramatic change in their life-styles.

Executives who want to effectively control their weight must do precisely that—adopt a *lifelong* weight-management program. That typically means a clearheaded assessment of how they gained the weight in the first place, followed by a specific plan for how they can realistically change their daily life-style for the rest of their lives. For virtually every executive, the plan involves increased exercise—the most effective way to permanently tip the calorie balance in your favor.

NUTRITION AND CANCER

A tremendous amount has been written about the links between food and cancer—both foods and dietary practices that might cause cancer—and nutrition as a way of preventing cancer. Although the data are far from perfect, there is enough concern in the medical and scientific community that in 1984 the American Cancer Society issued a special report titled "Nutrition and Cancer: Cause and Prevention." While the report did state that there is good evidence to suspect that dietary habits

93

may contribute to some forms of human cancer, it is important to be very cautious about leaping to cause-and-effect relationships.

There are, however, a few nutritional precautions that make sense, including avoiding obesity and decreasing your total fat intake. Increasing the amount of fiber in your diet and including foods high in vitamin A (typically dark green and deep yellow vegetables) and vitamin C (many fruits and vegetables) make sense. In addition to the other obvious health hazards of heavy alcohol consumption, it has been linked to an increased risk of cancers of the liver and esophagus.

In contrast to these rather straightforward precautions for reducing the likelihood of cancer, when it comes to the treatment of established cancer, there is no recognized value of any nutritional therapy. From time to time fads and extravagant claims arise for megavitamin or "natural food" therapies for cancer, but there is no valid scientific basis for these claims.

NUTRITION FOR ATHLETES

Many top executives remain interested in competitive athletics and are curious about how to modify their diets as well as evaluate some of the nutritional claims for various foods. In general, the principles of sound nutrition for athletes are the same as those of sound nutrition for anyone. Despite extravagant claims to the contrary, there is no convincing scientific evidence that most people can improve athletic performance by modifying a sound nutritional diet. There are a few minor exceptions.

The main problem, as I see it, is that many executives are functioning on information supplied to them by "the old coach" back in their college days in the 1950s and 1960s. In our survey, 77% of executives were competitive athletes in high school and 46% continued to compete in intercollegiate athletics. Clearly these individuals have carried their competitive spirit and determination forward into their business careers. Unfortunately, all too frequently they have also carried nutritional beliefs and habits based on outdated information into their adult athletic lives. Executives have described to me increasing the amount of protein in their diets during periods of intense training, eating a candy bar prior to a tennis match for "extra energy," and gulping salt tablets following intense bouts of exercise to "replace salt."

The idea that you need to increase your protein intake during athletic

94

training used to be ingrained in many college athletic programs. Its most notable manifestation was the famous pregame meal centered around a big steak. Even when this practice was most prevalent, there were no data to support it. Now we know that if you want to enhance performance during heavy training periods, the only modification that makes any sense is to slightly increase the amount of carbohydrates in your diet.

For most individuals, the best advice is simply to make sure that you are complying with the AHA guidelines of consuming 55% of your calories as carbohydrates. For elite college, professional, or Olympic endurance athletes, boosting the percentage of carbohydrates even a little further appears to make sense.

Should you load up on carbohydrates? This practice, where the amount of carbohydrates in the diet is transiently raised to around 70% of total calories, does make sense prior to a long endurance competition such as a marathon, but has no real role for the average adult even during vigorous training. The reason that "carbo-loading" seems to work prior to marathons is that it allows the muscles to become temporarily "supersaturated" with glycogen, which is the main fuel burned during prolonged endurance activity. If you wish to carbo-load, do it only for two or three days prior to an endurance competition and no more than two or three times a year.

There is probably no more important rule about nutrition during exercise than increasing fluid intake during periods of exertion. It used to be thought that you shouldn't drink fluids during exercise. This is absolutely *false* and potentially dangerous. Fortunately, every marathon competition is now required to provide water stations every two to three miles, and runners are strongly encouraged to drink the water. Yet, I still play tennis with executives who refuse to drink water during a match even during the hottest weather because of the mistaken belief that it will impair performance.

Nothing could be further from the truth. What *is* likely to impair performance is becoming dehydrated. Furthermore, thirst is a poor indicator of your body's need for fluid. You should make it a practice to pause to take in fluids (at least a six-ounce glass) every 15 minutes while exercising.

The drink of choice? Water! None of the so-called performance drinks has shown any significant benefit for the average athlete performing typical recreational sports lasting less than two hours. Some of the high-sugar drinks may actually be detrimental because they can impair fluid absorption and delay emptying of the stomach.

Salt tablets are another relic of the past. Popular in the 1950s and 1960s to replace salt lost during exercise and to "prevent cramps" (they don't work!), ingestion of salt tablets can actually be dangerous because it can lead to dehydration.

The final myth from the past is the sugar load prior to or during competition. As already noted, the ingestion of a candy bar leads to a transient rise of blood sugar, quickly followed by an outpouring of insulin from the pancreas, which leaves blood sugar unchanged or even lower.

The bottom line for the executive who wants to "eat to win" is to follow sound human nutrition in your daily life and drink plenty of water when you're exercising. The largest number of calories should be consumed at breakfast, followed by a moderate lunch and light supper. The reverse process, unfortunately all too common, is both an invitation to obesity and a setup for poor performance and lack of energy during the day.

DO-IT-YOURSELF TEST FOR WEIGHT CONTROL

One good way to estimate your desirable weight involves simple arithmetic.

FOR MEN
1. Record the number of inches in your height over 5' and multiple this number by 6.
2. Add 106. (Example: For a man who is 5'11" tall, $11'' \times 6 = 66 + 106 = 172$ pounds is ideal weight.)
3. Now weigh yourself.
4. Divide by your ideal weight to get your % over or under ideal weight. (Example: For a man who is 5'11" tall and weighs 200 pounds, $200/172 = 1.16$.) This man is 16% over ideal weight.

FOR WOMEN
1. Record the number of inches in your height over 5' and multiply this number by 5.
2. Add 100. (Example: For a woman who is 5'6" tall, $6'' \times 5 = 30 + 100 = 130$ pounds is ideal weight.)

3. Now weigh yourself.
4. Divide by your ideal weight to get your % over or under ideal weight. (Example: For a woman who is 5'6" tall and weighs 110 pounds, 110/130 = .85.) This woman is 85% of ideal weight, or 15% underweight.

How to rate your percent over ideal weight:

WEIGHT	RATING
At ideal body weight	Excellent
1–10% over ideal weight	Good
11–20% over ideal weight	Average
21–30% over ideal weight	Poor
31% or more over ideal weight	Very poor

5

Managing Stress

One of the most important attributes of a successful executive is the ability to cope with stress. I've seen a lot of people with tremendous ability who simply couldn't deal with stress. And those people, no matter how much ability they have, will always remain technicians at best. They never learn to live with the fact that their everyday decisions affect thousands of lives.

—ROBERT ROWAN, chairman and former CEO
Fruehauf

Executive stress. More has been written on this topic in the past five years than on almost any other issue related to executives' health. Business and medical journals are replete with stories about "executive burnout" and the physical and emotional travails of the "workaholic." Stress reduction programs have become part of the standard bill of fare in corporate wellness programs.

Our understanding of stress, how to recognize it and its physical and emotional consequences, has grown considerably in the past decade. Most current stress literature has one major shortcoming, however—it is based primarily on the observations of middle managers and does not apply to the senior-level executives represented in our survey. In fact, very little is known about stresses at the top of the corporate ladder, and the reason is simple: Senior executives are relatively inaccessible.

In our interviews and survey of CEOs, no subject aroused more interest than the issue of executive stress. The results provide new perspectives on the image of the overburdened executive constantly threatened with "burnout." When asked how much job-related pressure they usually experience, 53% of the executives responded "quite a bit" and 17% indicated "an extreme amount." Yet when asked the more salient question of how much negative job-related stress they usually experience, a much lower 30% responded "quite a bit" and only 5% replied "an extreme amount." Forty-seven percent indicated a "moderate amount" of negative stress and 18% "very little."

This suggests that top executives are confident of their ability to handle stress. A hefty 77% feel that they cope "very well" with job-related stresses; 21% think they handle it "fairly well"; and less than 2% think they do "poorly."

The portrait that emerges is a group of high-powered executives who experience pressure but who have learned to live with it and even thrive on it. They are what researchers would call "contented hard workers" rather than harried workaholics. With striking regularity the executives we interviewed emphasized that one of the prerequisites for their job was the ability to handle pressure without feeling overly stressed. Many described a winnowing process, a kind of corporate social Darwinism, in which those endowed with a higher tolerance for stress arrive at the executive suites. In fact, the ability to handle stress is as important, if not more important, than native managerial ability in rising to the top and functioning effectively once there.

Robert Rowan of Fruehauf related the following story: "Unfortunately, I recently had to make an executive change. . . . The guy had become very withdrawn, a loner, and had lost his ability to communicate. I've seen the many things that stress can do, and all of us react differently to it. Those who are able to cope with it are the ones who in the long run will be the most successful." Paul Allaire, president of Xerox Corporation, echoed a similar view: "The people who succeed are the people who handle stress on an ongoing basis without it bothering them—without it affecting their health and without it affecting their judgment."

This is not to suggest that chief executives are immune to stress. On the contrary, many are very candid about different sources of stress and strategies they have developed to deal with it throughout their careers. Most notable is a strong sense of experience and perspective and a great deal of pride in their acceptance of and ability to handle the day-to-day pressures of their jobs. The comments of Simon & Schuster's Richard Snyder are typical: "A CEO, if he has a good day, has fifty-one victories and thirty-one defeats. After the thirty-first time you get kicked in the stomach with something that didn't work out, you deal with it and go on to the next issue. I have so many decisions to make and so many things to deal with—both good and bad—I can't sit here and build up stress.

Sure, if we had a disaster, I'd feel stress. But in the normal course of business, I am so attuned to it and have dealt with it so long, as most CEOs have, that I don't feel stressed."

MANIFESTATIONS OF STRESS

What is stress and what is its impact on executive health and performance? In his landmark book *The Stress of Life*, published in 1956, Canadian scientist Hans Selye alerted people to the causes of stress and how it affects us physically and emotionally. Selye defined stress as "the nonspecific response of the body to any demand made upon it." The response is generalized—with both physical and mental components—and the demands may be internal or external.

For many years prior to Selye's work, neurophysiologists understood that a part of the nervous system supervises protective and housekeeping details in the human body in an automatic fashion. This portion of the nervous system is called "autonomic" to emphasize its automatic nature as opposed to the "voluntary" portion that is under your command. The autonomic nerve network is further divided into the "sympathetic" portion, which protects the body from danger, and the parasympathetic portion, which controls daily maintenance functions such as digestion, breathing, and heart rate at rest.

Harvard physiologist Walter Cannon characterized the sympathetic system as responsible for the capacity of "fright, fight, or flight" and the parasympathetic system as responsible for the functions of "rest and digest." It is when the former system responds to demands on the mind or body that many of the symptoms of stress occur.

A well-developed sympathetic nervous system had great adaptive value for our caveman ancestors. When confronted by a woolly mammoth, the caveman had to be able to experience instant fright and make the snap decision whether to stay and fight or take immediate flight. Those without superior sympathetic nervous systems, unable to put themselves on immediate full alert, simply didn't survive.

Thus, by the immutable law of survival of the fittest, we all inherit nervous systems capable of going on red alert with the slightest provocation. This would be perfectly reasonable if we spent our time dodging woolly mammoths, but it is highly dysfunctional when the major conflict is confrontation with other executives and subordinates. A pounding heartbeat, sweaty palms, and a feeling of edginess are all triggered by chemicals (largely adrenaline) from the sympathetic nervous system tricked into thinking that the stresses and strains of daily living constitute life-threatening emergencies requiring "fright, fight, or flight."

An important corollary to the physiologic response is the relationship between performance and stress. In 1908, Robert Yerkes and John Dodson, working at Harvard University's Physiologic Laboratory, described what is known as the "Yerkes-Dodson Law." According to this law, the relationship between stress and performance is a bell-shaped curve.

Below a certain level of stress, there are inadequate stimuli to solicit top performance. At certain levels of stress, outstanding performance is elicited. When stress exceeds this level, however, performance trails off rapidly.

In one way or another, virtually every executive we interviewed believes in this relationship—both in their own capacities and those of their subordinates. One CEO described a vice-president who had performed flawlessly until he reached a senior management level. Once there, the executive's work began to decline, and he finally had to be terminated. It turned out that he had been accomplishing increasingly difficult jobs by working longer hours. Once promoted above a certain level, he simply ran out of time and the stress overwhelmed him.

Among the executives we interviewed, there is no doubt that an individual's performance zone can be expanded or altered, and, in fact, a great deal of their time is devoted to determining the right levels for their managers. "According to the Peter Principle, people get promoted until they reach a level where they don't have the skills to handle a job. I've seen people promoted to their level of incompetence. *But* the incompetence comes from the fact that their new responsibilities are imposing more stress on them than they have the capability to handle," observed William Coors. "I've been trying—and one day I'll succeed—to measure the stress quotient in any individual. That way, if his job puts him at the top level of what you might call constructive stress, you know damn well not to increase his load or you're going to cause tremendous problems."

While the relationship between stress and performance is accepted by most experts, the links between stress and a variety of medical problems are given much less credence. Many of these possible links are hotly debated in the medical community. The gamut of medical problems—some minor and some life-threatening—thought to be stress related runs from cardiovascular disease to psychosomatic disorders.

STRESS AND THE HEART

The important connections between head and heart are only slowly coming to light. There has always been a folklore of tragic heroes and heroines who "died of a broken heart," and in cardiology we have come to realize that there are some situations where life truly does imitate art.

Perhaps the most famous theory linking stress to heart disease was formulated by Drs. Meyer Friedman and Ray H. Rosenman in their concept of "Type A behavior." Their theory, which is frequently misinterpreted, describes the behavior of individuals (typically men) who see their lives as a constant struggle. Type A people feel trapped in an unremitting drive to accomplish more and more in less and less time. Their drive is typically accompanied by, and undercut by, excessive urgency, intolerance for delay, hostility, and hyperaggressive competitiveness. This behavior pattern was first identified in a study of Friedman's and Rosenman's cardiac patients who had suffered heart attacks.

Unfortunately, many people associate "Type A" with hard working, aggressive individuals, and fail to recognize the unhappy compulsive behavior that characterizes the true "A" person. Indeed, some individuals proudly label themselves "Type A" in the context of a Red Badge of Courage, seemingly unaware of the misery of the full-blown syndrome.

Friedman and Rosenman made a compelling case, subsequently corroborated by other investigators, that individuals who experience life as constant stress expose themselves to a marked increase in the likelihood of developing coronary heart disease (CHD).

Other cardiovascular symptoms, such as an increase in the heart rate, have been linked to stress as well. We have all experienced the sensation of our hearts racing before a speech or presentation. That is nothing more than the sympathetic nervous system getting us ready for "fright, fight, or flight." The process can lead to extra heartbeats—ventricular premature beats, or "VPBs" in medical parlance—that range from benign palpitations to severe rhythm problems that can even occasionally result in sudden cardiac arrest. In the latter, the heart begins to beat so chaotically that it can no longer effectively pump blood. Unless instant action is taken to restore normal cardiac rhythm, the victim collapses and dies.

While stress is an unusual cause of sudden death, it can be severe enough to cause the heartbeat to degenerate rapidly. There are well-documented cases of individuals whose heartbeats become chaotic when they are exposed to psychological stress. In fact, the incidence is common enough that one group of cardiologists in Boston who specialize in rhythm disorders include psychological testing as a routine part of pretreatment evaluations.

Stress may also cause cardiovascular false alarms. I have treated a number of executives for chest pains they thought to be impending heart attacks that turned out to be manifestations of stress. One CEO of a manufacturing company was experiencing chest pains during or shortly after emotional periods, such as arguments at work or home. A vigorous man in his mid-forties, he regularly played strenuous singles tennis and jogged three times a week. He had never smoked or had high blood pressure, and his cholesterol was only slightly elevated at 220 mg/dl. There was no history of heart disease in his family. His appointment was prompted by an incident the previous afternoon at work. He had had a heated discussion with a senior vice-president, after which he experienced several brief shooting pains in his chest when he returned to his office.

Even though the likelihood of CHD was very low, he was given a complete physical examination, an electrocardiogram, and an exercise tolerance test, all of which were entirely normal. It was evident that this CEO was suffering from stress that manifested itself as chest pain. As it turned out, six months earlier the company that he had built from scratch went public. While the stock offering had been successful, the entire rules of the game had changed. Before, when he owned the company, if he had a good idea he simply went out and implemented it. Now there were stockholders and money managers, and he viewed his job as "one long series of compromises." The situation was much more stressful than he had realized, and the chest pains were the result of that stress.

After reassuring this young executive that I had found no evidence of CHD, we discussed the types of stress he was experiencing. He was relieved by the findings of the electrocardiogram and exercise test and resolved to take more structured breaks, such as daily exercise, to keep his work and stress levels in perspective.

There are two points to this story. First, stress can bring on a variety of physical symptoms, including chest pains that may resemble angina or a heart attack. This is not uncommon. In our Heart Catheterization Laboratory at the University of Massachusetts Medical Center, for example, about 10% of the patients we catheterize for chest pain symptoms prove to have normal coronary arteries. Stress is undoubtedly playing a role in many, if not most, of these cases.

Second—and most important—the onset of chest pains of any kind should always be taken seriously, and anyone who experiences them should consult a cardiologist as soon as possible.

STRESS AND THE MIND

The effects of stress are by no means confined to the heart and cardiovascular system. Indeed, the most pervasive impact of stress on executives relates to mental health. The branch of medical science that focuses on the links between mind states and physical ailments is called psychosomatic medicine. In certain areas, such as the link between stress and headaches, the connection is well established, although the exact mechanism is still debated. In our survey, 29% of the respondents listed at least one physical symptom that they attributed to stress. Mirroring a smaller poll conducted in 1982 for the *Wall Street Journal,* headaches led our list. Other manifestations of executive stress may range from fatigue and sleeplessness to full-blown, career-threatening depression.

One CEO of an entrepreneurial firm reported that he was experiencing stomach pains as a result of the "tremendous pressure" he felt trying to build the business. Few of the executives we interviewed, however, reported severe physical problems, although all admitted to periods of fatigue and occasional insomnia usually tied to a specific incident or circumstance.

"There are times when stress gets very high, particularly when we are in dangerous financial circumstances, and I wake up at three o'clock in the morning," admitted one CEO. "Often the solution just involves taking some action the next day that any fool is capable of. But at three A.M., just lying there with the problem can be very depressing. Fortunately, it doesn't happen very often—I've experienced it only three or four times."

At its worst, stress can lead to isolation and depression of career- or even life-threatening proportions. Writing in the *Wall Street Journal* about his own depression, James Turner, a former CEO, stated:

> Executives and managers, especially those high on the organizational chart, are particularly vulnerable to depression. Higher equates with lonelier; self-protection dictates one can't unburden one's emotional weakness with subordinates or competitive peers—or anyone else for that matter. The ultimate in emotional isolation is the chief executive. He can display no weakness, admit to no doubt or fear, and few, if any, subordinates would dare broach the subject of his mental well-being with him.

Such isolation can ultimately immobilize the normally action-oriented chief executive, as Turner recounted:

> My own depression, much like the tropical kind that grows into a hurricane, began to increase in intensity in the last couple of months. Looking back, I can even see a distinct change in my signature. There had been a gradual but accelerating change in my relation to my associates and subordinates, characterized by my withdrawal. I began to feel that all communications, regardless of content, were negative, and through association turned these feelings toward the bearer. Peer contacts, generally lunches with CEOs of other companies, which I enjoyed at least twice monthly, trickled to a halt. As I withdrew further, I became reluctant to call the necessary management meetings.

Turner's depression ultimately resulted in the loss of his job, but enabled him to seek the help he needed. While certainly not all depression is attributable to stress, the two are often closely related.

The mental effects of stress are well established and seldom debated. New frontiers in psychosomatic medicine, however, are pushing into some areas that were previously thought to be entirely physical. Research now shows that some diseases, including cancer, may have a component of stress. While we are a long way from definitive cures for most forms of cancer, medical science is beginning to explain how normal cells may be transformed into invasive cancer cells. Until recently, little credence was given to the role of emotion and stress in cancer. In one study, conducted by the U.S. Navy, captains who were passed over for promotion to rear admiral had a dramatic increase in the incidence of cancer in the next year. Coincidence? Perhaps.

Stress may also contribute to joint inflammation and arthritis. In one study of workers whose plant was threatened with closing, the incidence of inflamed joints rose dramatically then just as quickly declined when the corporation decided to keep the plant open.

One explanation of the link between stress and these medical problems may involve the immune system. This system comprises the body's main defense against infection and, to some degree, cancers. Disruption of the immune system can leave an individual susceptible to a variety of problems possibly ranging from more colds to less ability to resist cancer.

SOURCES OF STRESS

While the results of our survey show that top executives have a high tolerance for stress, distinct patterns emerge when levels of executive stress are analyzed by type of company. Most interesting, but not surprising, is that the top executives in entrepreneurial firms—those on the *Inc.* 100 and *Venture* lists—report higher degrees of job-related pressure and negative stress than their counterparts in the larger, well-established *Fortune* 500 companies. For example, while 82% of the respondents from the *Inc.* and *Venture* lists experience "quite a bit" or an "extreme amount" of work pressure, a significantly lower 60% from the *Fortune* list fall in those categories, with those managing Dun's large and small companies falling between these extremes (71%). The corresponding figures for negative stress show a similar pattern: 36% of the *Inc.* and *Venture* executives report significant amounts of negative stress, compared with 27% of the *Fortune* 500 executives. The entrepreneurs are also less sanguine about their ability to handle job-related stress, with 37% claiming to cope very well versus 48% for the *Fortune* executives.

In our interviews, executives from both entrepreneurial enterprises and the older, well-established firms—some of whom had worked for both types of operations—offered a number of explanations for the differences in stress levels. Personal and corporate financial concerns are one of the major culprits. For most of the *Fortune* 500 executives, personal financial security is no longer an issue, and although the financial performance of their companies can be a worry, the risks and repercussions of day-to-day decisions are nowhere near as immediate. For the entrepreneurs, on the other hand, financial issues are the primary source of stress. Avner Parnes, former chairman and CEO of MBI Business Centers, described a common problem: "The pressure in raising money is tremendous. You believe in your product, but nobody believes in you. When they finally give you some limited resources, they throw a lot of obstacles in your way. All of these things put more and more pressure on you. There's constant pressure from the bank to sell more. In addition, you've probably risked a lot of your own money. So you're at the tip of the pyramid, with nobody to show you how to handle those things. It's very, very tough."

Several *Inc.* and *Venture* CEOs described the financial pressures of their early years in particular. "I left a lucrative job to go out and risk everything," noted Terry Jacobs, chairman of Jacor Communications. "I borrowed as much money as I could and took all of the equity I had accumulated and bet it on this new company. My kids were in high school or younger, and the thing that worried me the most was whether I would be able to provide them with the education they would need. That was probably the greatest worry."

The ability to withstand this kind of stress—betting everything on a new venture—in part defines the entrepreneur. And while they are quick to acknowledge the strains, many thrive in their environment. "Becoming a public company has been a lot of fun for us, for me in particular," explained Dr. Leonard Reiffel, CEO of Interand. "I enjoy, most of the time at least, coping with the pressures of trying to explain our goals to the investment community, financial community, and our shareholders. It's a real challenge."

The financial pressures on CEOs and presidents of large companies are different from those of entrepreneurs, but no less real. The tenure of a senior manager can turn on the ability to meet budgets and maintain a certain level of profitability. "The biggest source of stress is when you're not making budget, when your numbers are no good," confided Lin Patterson, president and CEO of Appleton & Lange. "You have to figure out if there is anything you can do about it, or if it's only timing or whatever. Then you have to decide how you're going to present the situation to the rest of management."

To some extent, the differences in attitudes and practices between *Inc./Venture* executives and *Fortune* 500 CEOs may be attributable as much to age as to differences in the work environment. On average, the *Inc.* and *Venture* executives are 45, almost a decade younger than their

107

Fortune counterparts, at 54. Another decade of experience and proven job security apparently changes the way executives of the largest companies view the world and their own priorities.

In many ways, the pressures on rising entrepreneurs are similar to those experienced by intensely competitive younger managers in larger companies trying to make their mark as they rise through company ranks. It's the drive to succeed, whether against others in the market or others in the company. In fact, with few exceptions, the *Fortune* 500 executives we interviewed agree that there was much more stress earlier in their careers than there is at the top. As one CEO put it: "On the way up, a considerable source of pressure is competition—some of it to become CEO. Technically, once you've reached the top, you don't have that competition anymore. You're king of the hill. But on the way up, you're vying against five or ten other guys."

Once at the top, as many CEOs pointed out, their responsibilities and sources of stress change. "The earlier stresses were different," explained Tenneco chairman and CEO J. L. Ketelsen. "The one stress that you don't have as a CEO is the stress that a boss can create. You eliminate that side of the stress equation that middle management has. Your board of directors is there and that creates new pressures, but that's not the same thing as working for a boss who's riding you day in and day out.

"The obvious thing, though, is when you get done with it, you're responsible for the final decisions and all the key results. Granted, a lot of people are involved, but the buck stops with you and that does create a high level of responsibility and whatever stress comes with it."

For the entrepreneur out on a limb, often by himself, that high level of responsibility can be extremely stressful. "The pressure is just tremendous. There's definitely pressure on the people who work for you, but it's much less than it is on you," said MBI's Avner Parnes. "You're the one who signs the notes and loans. You're the one whose name appears on everything, and you're the one responsible to the investor."

A common source of concern among CEOs is the responsibility they feel for their employees. "A person at the top of the management hierarchy is theoretically responsible for everybody on down. And you can let those responsibilities weigh heavily on you; you get seriously concerned about the welfare of your people. A company's success depends on the performance of its people, and it takes ten thousand people to run a company like this," explained William Coors. "You have to have teamwork to get the job done. There are those constant anxieties. You get involved where the system isn't perfect, all the little flaws come to attention. Somebody isn't happy; this happened or that happened. So there's constant pressure."

Perhaps the most stressful people-management situation for executives is when a substantial cutback in personnel must be made. Donald Lennox, who was brought in to save the failing International Harvester, described the situation he faced when he became CEO: "We had to take extremely unpleasant actions to survive and, as we closed plants, we became acutely aware of the devastating effect we were having on peoples' lives, their families, and communities. You can't just walk away from people; you can't just shut down operations and merrily dismiss workers and officers of the company. . . . The only way I did what I had to do was to keep reassuring myself that we were taking the only course of action available to us."

Dismissals of other members of senior management are particularly stressful. As Tenneco's J. L. Ketelsen explained, describing the cutbacks his company had to make following a plunge in oil prices: "It was the first significant cutback the company had ever had, and it created a lot of extra stress at the top of the organization, where we took out fifteen percent to twenty percent of our people, including senior management. It's something you don't want to do, but there's no choice when you're in a situation where the price of your product drops sixty percent in three months. . . . It is very, very difficult, particularly when you have to tell a person face-to-face that his job has been phased out. It's the hardest thing you have to do as an executive in terms of emotional strain."

Donald Lennox provided a similar example of how hard this process was during the downsizing of Navistar: "I knew one afternoon that I was going to have to inform some senior executives that their jobs had been eliminated. You have to do a certain amount of psyching up as you get ready to bring them in. When I told them, they were extremely distressed. Some cried, or pleaded for a chance to do anything. But I knew the decision had been made and no compromise was possible. It's a very emotionally unpleasant experience."

On the other side of the coin are problems associated with promotions. "I've been in a number of stressful situations where I've had to make some really tough personal decisions and I've had to let some people go. More frequently, though, the kind of stress I've confronted is where I had to promote one person and not somebody else—and deal with the person who didn't get promoted or with his wife," recalled one senior vice-president.

The pressures associated with negotiating critical business deals are also a source of stress, particularly when there are unanticipated hurdles. "When we bought Houston Oil and Minerals back in 1981, it was a very big acquisition, and it came about the time oil prices were starting to break," explained Tenneco's former executive vice-president Joe B. Foster. "As we got into head-to-head negotiations, we ran into a number of things we didn't expect when we initiated the deal. Trying to sort out all the problems that arose created real stress. Other deals have created a certain amount of stress, but that one was the one time in my career I felt completely stressed out."

Wheeling and dealing can represent even greater risk taking for entrepreneurs, and with it can come significantly greater stress. As MCI's Donald Steen pointed out, "Ours is a developing business and, dealing with physicians in thirty-five locations, it's not a stable business. If the plastic surgeons in Houston got mad at us, they could put us right out of business in that city if they wanted to. So there's a constant stress from that viewpoint. Everything's going great on Monday. Then on Tuesday you have major problems in three different centers. Maybe three years from now when our company is bigger and more successful, it won't be such a big deal. But these concerns are a major deal now."

Perhaps the most universal source of stress for executives is the extraordinary demands placed on their time. "Most of my stress comes when I'm in a hurry, when I have ten things to do and nine time slots available," noted Xerox's Paul Allaire. "It's tough just to say, 'OK, time out, I'm going to take a few minutes to relax, or I'm going to go for a walk around the corridors.' You tend not to do that when you need it the most."

However, the bottom-line source of stress—the one mentioned most frequently by top executives—is yourself. "An awful lot of managers create stresses and strains all by themselves," observed John Bierwirth, senior management consultant and former chairman and CEO of Grumman Corp. "It's just human nature, I'm afraid. I try to teach junior executives to relax with the facts as they are and not get tense over the fact that it's snowing, so to speak, because there's not a damn thing they can do about it."

"Once you know what you're bucking, don't turn it on yourself. That's what creates stress. You put stress on yourself; no one else can put it on you," added Fruehauf's Robert Rowan.

Top executives admit that it is frustrating to watch senior managers crumble under stress they create for themselves. The president of a *Fortune* 500 company described such a situation: "We have one executive who is very good, but who is as wound-up as any person I know. He was that way when he had a key operations job, so we moved him into a corporate staff position. That should have been a lot more relaxing, but it only made matters worse—because he doesn't have as much control, I guess.

"So it's not the environment that puts stress on this guy. He puts it on himself."

STRATEGIES FOR MANAGING STRESS

Most of this book is about strategies—programs to help executives keep body and soul together in their unique environments. Not surprisingly, most of those we interviewed had definite philosophies and methods for handling stress. Although their approaches differ, a few underlying themes emerge. The first is the recognition that, regardless of the degree to which it is felt and the way in which it is handled, stress is a constant factor in their daily jobs.

"I've spent an awful lot of time thinking about stresses and how to eliminate them from the job, and I've come to the conclusion that you can't," noted William Coors. "You can eliminate people stress—you can eliminate friction between people. But as far as the day-to-day anxiety of whether this product is selling or isn't selling and the other problems you have, you can't eliminate those stresses. What you have to do is to learn how to handle them."

Furthermore, Coors and his counterparts strongly believe that coping with stress is a personal, individual matter. "You have to have a system for keeping things in perspective and controlling the major stresses in your own life," asserted Xerox's Allaire. "Everyone has his own approach to managing stress. If you didn't, you wouldn't be able to succeed because you wouldn't have the clarity of mind and physical stamina to keep at it."

Reflected in the individualistic approach to stress management is a high degree of skepticism about formal stress-reduction programs. "If people feel the need for a program, we have it available to them. But I think it's an individual problem; most stress-reduction programs are really a waste of time. Everybody's got to cope with their own problems in their own way. The same way I feel that religion is a personal preference, I feel that health and stress is a personal matter," explained one CEO.

This is not to suggest that CEOs are unaware of, or unsympathetic to, the problems of stress among executives and other employees in their organizations. While they feel that formal stress-reduction programs don't work for them, many have established in-house or referral services for employees who feel they need professional help.

Among the strategies for managing stress, the key factors most frequently mentioned are physical well-being and mental outlook. Unquestionably, exercise is the most common source of relief. In our survey, "stress reduction" was one of the major reasons respondents cited for their exercise programs.

A number of recent scientific studies have shown the connection between vigorous exercise and mental benefits. A study at the University of Massachusetts Medical School Physiology Laboratory extended these findings to a relatively less vigorous form of exercise—walking at various speeds. In a series of workouts, 36 volunteers between ages 30 and 50 were asked to walk on a treadmill for 40 minutes at various paces. A battery of psychological tests was used to measure their anxiety, tension, and mood before, during, and after the walks. The results showed that walking at even a slow speed produced significant reductions in anxiety and tension and improvements in mood. As an added physical bonus, the walkers also experienced a significant reduction in their blood pressure that lasted for up to two hours after their walks.

The experience of the executives in our survey corroborate such findings. The following statements are typical of their attitudes toward exercise.

From Tenneco's K. W. Reese: "There's no question that my exercise program has helped me cope with stress. I've learned that if stress builds up, I just go out and run like hell. I'm a morning runner and that sets the tone for the whole day. By the time I get to the office, I'm relaxed. I feel good."

Terry Jacobs of Jacor Communications: "If I go for a week without exercising—say I've been sick or something's come up that I haven't been able to exercise—I feel the difference mentally. Exercise has definitely played a great role in my ability to cope with stress and keep it in the right perspective."

Simon & Schuster's Richard Snyder: "I exercise in a utilitarian manner. It's not a philosophical point for me. I use it to reduce stress and free my mind. I've learned to use it on problems that seem impossible and to use it on a bad day. I feel a hundred percent better when I finish. It's a physical difference."

Fruehauf's Rowan is so committed to exercise for stress reduction that he constructed a small workout room adjacent to his executive suite for use by his entire senior staff: "We discuss it from time to time and everybody agrees that exercise is the best way to alleviate stress," he explained. "When things build up to a point, you should do something physically—and that reduces the mental strains and stresses. It's pretty hard for a tired body to feel anything but good."

Many executives use daily periods of exercise as much for creative thinking time away from pressures as for relaxing tension.

MCI's Donald Steen commented: "When I don't feel good, it's often hard to tell if it is stress related or lack of exercise. I do find that exercise helps a lot. It's so nice in the morning to plan your day while you're running. You can think through problems; things that may have been fuzzy the night before become clearer to me when I've been exercising."

Coors Vice-President of Sales and Marketing Bob Rechholtz, who exercises in Colorado's outdoors during most of the year, agreed: "It's new scenery, fresh air, and no phones—the natural environment helps relieve stress. I think about business when I'm working out, but in a much more creative manner because I'm physically relaxed and my mind is cleared to operate without interruptions. I come up with a lot of solutions to tough problems when I'm exercising."

CEOs also welcome competitive forms of exercise as opportunities to take their minds completely off business matters. Concentrating on a vigorous tennis game, serious golf match, or challenging downhill ski run against the clock, for example, provides valuable mental "time-outs."

"When you're serving for set and match point or trying to sink a birdie putt on the eighteenth, you're not thinking about anything else," said Tenneco's Joe B. Foster, an active tennis player. "And when you're finished, you know you've had the type of break you really needed."

Among individual strategies for stress management, the most pervasive is a strong emphasis on accepting the facts of a situation. Talking about a particularly stressful period at Nashua Corporation, when he had to lay off senior management people, Charles Clough noted, "It's very tough. For many of them, it wasn't their fault that things didn't work out. . . . Whenever you have to do something like that, you just have to work it through, making certain that you have all the facts and that you have no other alternative."

Similarly, Donald Lennox described how he approached the downsizing of Navistar by learning to live with the reality of the situation. "I approached it on the basis that I was working hard night and day, thinking about every possible alternative and getting as much consultation as I could from the staff on the best courses of action. If in the end, we wound up failing and the whole thing went down the tube, I could look at myself in the mirror and say, 'Well, it wasn't because you were playing golf or horsing around. You really did your best.' That saved me from becoming a dishrag or losing sleep.

"The biggest mistake anybody in this type of job can make is to try to do it all alone. You have to be willing to reach out. And to do that, you have to admit that you don't have all the answers," added Lennox.

Another common approach to dealing with potentially stressful situations is to follow Satchel Paige's advice: "Don't look back. Something may be gaining on you." As Tenneco's J. L. Ketelsen commented, "It helps to be forward oriented and not dwell on the past. You have to look back, analyze mistakes, and learn from them. But you can create an awful lot of stress by worrying about what you've done. It's a lot more constructive and a lot less stressful to plan for the future than to worry about what you did wrong, what you might have done, or what you didn't do in the past."

A specific strategy for jettisoning stress from past events was offered by EG&G's Dean Freed: "If something is preying on you for more than twenty-four hours, you have to develop a scheme where you can put it on the shelf. You might not be able to make it go away, but you have to get on with life. You can't let it gnaw away at you."

Planning ahead as much as possible is an effective tactic for minimizing stress, as Joe B. Foster found during the staff reductions at Tenneco.

"I had to talk to senior executives about early retirement, and we started with at least five or six months' notice," recalled Foster. "I talked with a fellow in March about retiring November first; in fact, I talked to him for three months before he said, 'You know, I really ought to retire.' It reinforced my whole theory about business—the fewer shocks, the better. By planning ahead, there are fewer surprises and with fewer surprises there's a lot less stress."

One of the most frequently mentioned ways to avoid stress is delegation. Almost all of the executives we interviewed had experienced situations where a senior manager had been promoted to a position with more responsibility but simply couldn't "let go" and delegate. The managers ended up crumbling under the strain of trying to deal personally with every problem that came their way. One CEO noted that the first question he asks a staff member who presents him with a problem is, "What do *you* recommend?" This has proven to be an effective tactic for getting subordinates to think issues through and present solutions or options rather than place the problem on his shoulders.

By far the most common advice top executives offer for dealing with stress—and perhaps the most difficult for junior executives to follow—is a conscientious effort to maintain a balanced perspective. As Ronald Thomas, chairman and former president of Ciprico, Inc., put it: "You have to make a conscious decision to put this much effort into family, this much effort into health, and this much into business. That should be something you give a lot of thought to—trying to balance it out." Echoed Xerox's Allaire, "You need to develop a balance between your intellectual life, your cultural life, your family life, your physical well-being, and your work life. You have to have a method for making the necessary trade-offs so that you don't let any one of those get out of proportion."

How do you maintain such a balance? Apart from physical exercise, periods of rest and structured time away from the office are extremely important. Many executives described how they had learned the hard way to simply take a break. "At some point, I finally recognized that you have to rest—whether that rest comes from taking a weekend and going to Florida or going to bed one night at ten o'clock. I realized that there is a fatigue factor, and you have to do something about it," said Allaire.

Most of the executives plan weekends and vacations where they are completely away and relatively inaccessible. "My idea of a vacation lately is the type you take with one or two other people and a radio that doesn't work. It's rafting on the Colorado River or going on a safari—where I can't be reached," explained Simon & Schuster's Snyder.

Planned "time-out" is easier said than done for some executives so attuned to constant contact with the office. "I always try to give myself a free day on the weekend. I'd rather work on Saturday and know that once I finish, the briefcase goes back on the desk and I'm free," noted Snyder. "Sometimes I can do that and sometimes I can't . . . but it's bullshit to say you need to call in all the time. A lot of guys just check in to make sure they're needed."

For Snyder and his counterparts, just getting physically away from the office is extremely important. "I have a house in the country which I generally go to on weekends. I'll leave the city around five o'clock and arrive by seven. . . . I'll get out of the suit, into a pair of blue jeans, have a vodka martini, play with the dog or go for a walk on the property. Within thirty minutes, I'm a different person," he confessed.

As individuals, the top executives have found ways to put their jobs in perspective. It can be as simple as taking a walk along a river, as Fruehauf's Robert Rowan observed. "All of us have to learn the things we can do to best live with stress," he said. "When I reach the point where I've just about had it, I know what I have to do to get back in perspective—get my thoughts and objectives back on those things that are really important. I love the outdoors. After a hard day, I just go out and walk along the river. To me, it brings back the perspective. No matter how important things are at the office, they pale next to that river. It's been flowing there for a thousand years and will flow for a thousand years more. What we do today in the big scheme of things is like a drop of rain during a rainstorm. It helps bring me back to the basic things like family and health, and all the things that are far more important than the problems I'm dealing with today."

THE TIES THAT BIND

As a group, the top executives in our survey have come to grips with pressures in their personal lives, much as they have done in their professional lives. When asked about levels of negative personal stress they experience, 85% indicated a moderate or very little amount. Only one of the 1,139 respondents replied an extreme amount. Similarly, in their ability to cope with personal stress, 70% feel they do well or very well and only 5% feel they do poorly.

What matters most to these top executives? What gives them the greatest personal satisfaction? Salary? Work? Investments? Sports? Not even close. When asked to rate the level of personal satisfaction they derive from a variety of factors in their lives, both personal and professional, the highest sources of satisfaction by a wide margin are family, spouse, and children. Work, sports, religion, hobbies, investments, and community work all score significantly lower.

Far too little has been written about the positive factors in executives' personal lives that counterbalance the pressures of top corporate jobs or the strains of launching an entrepreneurial enterprise. This is because most want it that way. Top executives may be highly visible at work, but they don't want to live in "glass houses" at home and purposefully shield their personal lives from public view. As one CEO put it: "I view my personal life as an oasis, a place to go for refreshment and regeneration. And I want to keep it that way."

Yet in the responses to our questionnaire and our interviews, the top executives were willing, and some even surprisingly eager, to share their personal lives and philosophies. One resounding message came through loud and clear: Business success is no substitute for personal happiness, and personal happiness is almost invariably tied to a happy and supportive family life. "It's hard for me to see how a man could ever be successful in a major corporation without a wife along as a partner, supporting him and being part of his efforts to achieve success," observed Robert Rowan. "Before I consider somebody for a high position, I make it a point to meet his family—just to evaluate the background he's coming from. I'm not saying that's the only criterion for a successful executive, but it makes it a lot easier."

"A good family life is critical," echoed Norton vice-president of human resources Thomas Hourihan. "The job isn't the place to escape from an unhappy personal situation. In fact, we have seen a number of cases where unhappy domestic situations had a direct impact on executive job performance. My family is tremendously important to me. I've never had to choose between business and family, but if a business decision meant diminishing my family life, I wouldn't do it."

The overwhelming majority—89%—of the executives in our survey were married. Approximately 6% were divorced or separated; 3% were single; and 1% widowed. Most of the executives we interviewed were happily married to their first wife or husband. Those who had gone through divorce or were separated uniformly cited the experience as the most severely stressful period in their lives. "The major source of stress in my life was my divorce. It came from personal, family problems, not work. If you want to make money, your next book should be how to get through divorce without stress!" advised one recently divorced CEO.

A few who had been divorced or widowed were happily remarried. "It's wonderful to be married to somebody who is supportive of your career. There's nothing like it," exclaimed one CEO. "I feel more mature in my current marriage than my previous one, where there was always a kind of harping. It's hard to go to work and be president of a company and come home and have somebody complaining all the time."

Fruehauf's Rowan considers himself equally lucky. "My first wife died twelve years ago, which was devastating for me. Some people say a man can't be lucky twice, but I was. I was remarried three years ago to a very wonderful lady who makes my life very complete. I think it would be awfully hard to cope with the stresses and strains I deal with if I couldn't look forward to going home and spending time with my family. They're far more important to me than any successes I've achieved in the business world."

The executives left little doubt about the role of the home as a harbor, an oasis, a source of support and deep personal ties. It is an essential element in their emotional health. You can almost feel the RPMs of the office winding down in the description provided by Interand's Leonard Reiffel. "There's a psychological mind-set that occurs. I'm fortunate in being very happily married. And what I find is that when I get into the car to go home and turn on the ignition, it's almost like operant conditioning. I can just feel the tension go. Obviously, there are times when this doesn't work, but ninety-five times out of a hundred when I go through the mental imagery of going home and seeing my wife, I can feel the tension go away. By the time I actually get home, it's like some of the extra switches have been turned off."

By no means, however, did these executives indicate that they lead stress-free personal lives. Many spoke candidly about the strains of balancing business and family demands, lamenting the toll that long hours take on their spouses and families, particularly in their earlier years climbing the corporate ladder or establishing their own busi-

118

nesses. "Being a CEO is the easy part; you have all those years of experience. It's getting there that's the hard part. That's where a lot of stress comes in," said one executive. "I think it's almost impossible to be a good husband and a striving thirty-year-old moving up the corporate ladder."

A number of executives looked back with wistfulness and regret to some of the choices they made in the early periods of their careers and the impact on their families. As one CEO explained: "In the early years there are some definite sacrifices from a family standpoint. Had I known when I started the degree of activity it would take to reach a certain level of success, I would have taken a little less success and spent more time with the family and less on the business."

Some of the top executives in entrepreneurial firms, in particular, vividly recall the personal strains associated with a start-up and the shock when they recognized the toll it was taking on their families. "I had thrown myself completely into the business. It had assumed priority over everything else—over family, kids, everything," explained one *Inc.* CEO. "I remember the exact date when it hit me what I was doing. It was August 15, 1981. I had bought the business two months before. I was living in a different city from my family, and I called home every day. My son answered the phone and in the conversation he said, 'Dad, do you know what day it is?' I said, 'Thursday.' He said, 'Dad, it's my birthday.'. . . Looking back, I even saw it happening. I just couldn't control it."

A happy home life for top executives isn't a given. Like anyone else, they have to work at it—perhaps harder. Many described how they had developed plans and schedules, which they rarely altered, to keep their professional responsibilities from overwhelming their family lives. The routine established by Paul Allaire and his wife, for example, was not uncommon. "You just have to make a decision and stick with it. And it helps to have a family who will hold you to it as much as the company does. For example, when we were in England, we lived in London but we also had a place in the country. On Friday night we went to the country and on Sunday we came home. I never took work with me, so the only way I could work on the weekends was when we got back to London Sunday night. We also made a decision to do something cultural every Wednesday night. I stuck to that religiously. I simply wouldn't schedule business meetings or accept invitations for Wednesday night."

In addition to weekends off and evenings out, family vacations are extremely important to top executives as a way of structuring personal retreats. No matter how busy, most of the executives lived up to a self-imposed commitment to take at least one week, and often more, away from the office since the earliest years of their careers. Some, like Federal-Mogul's T. F. Russell, consider it critical that a husband and wife get away periodically, too. "It's important to periodically stop and say, 'OK, we're going to take a three-day or five-day vacation together," advised Russell. "It's particularly important when you're raising young children. Even though you may not have the opportunity to be with your children, you have to provide the outlet for your wife to get away from that responsibility so the two of you can do whatever you want to do for a few days."

A common concern for time-pressed executives is staying in touch with their children and their activities. A supportive spouse understands missing a social obligation here and there. Children do not have the same perspective and often resent the fact that Dad or Mom missed the "Big Game," the band concert, or the ballet recital, because he or she had to "work late at the office." Again, the strategy employed by the top executives we interviewed is to make time for what is important to them and their families, to structure their schedules so that company demands do not completely erode their personal lives.

"It's been tough, but the family knows that I'm very engrossed in the business," explained Terry Jacobs. "I try to spend all day Sunday and at least one or two evenings a week in family get-togethers. We make it a point to let the children know that what they're involved in is very important to us. We haven't missed one of our sons' college football games in four-and-a-half years. Our daughter is involved in playing soccer and other activities. I put the games on my calendar and make it a point of being there. What's important to them is important to me."

If executives place demands on their families, they also find ways to try to compensate for it. Family celebrations, special trips, or evenings out are shared on many occasions. Here's how one entrepreneur described what he did the day his company went public and he received a check for several million dollars: "As a surprise, I hired a helicopter and flew my wife around New York that evening at sunset with a bottle of champagne and a couple of crystal glasses I bought at Tiffany's. I laid New York at her feet, romantic fool that I am. She loved it and I loved it. . . . I told the story to one of my investment guys on Wall Street and he said, 'You're going to convince me that you're one hell of a guy if you tell me that you threw those hundred-dollar champagne glasses out the window!' "

The support network constructed by executives usually extends beyond their families to a few close friends. But while such friendships are valuable, all of the executives were quick to point out that there is no substitute for those at home. Said one CEO: "I spend more of my time socializing with my family than I do with anybody else, and they appreciate it a lot more. If you take care of your family, they are always going to be there in good times or bad to help you. If you don't take care of them, it can be an awfully lonely, difficult life."

6

Optimizing Your Health and Fitness

I urge young executives to stay fit. Sit back sometimes and ask what you're doing and review it—very much like a business plan. Too much work? Too little play? What about my body weight and blood pressure? Take care of your mind and body. Exercise, eat right, control stress, and keep a positive attitude. Have a good time being idle and never underestimate the importance of friends and loved ones. . . . Choosing a life-style is ours for the asking—we get what we decide. We achieve what we make up our minds to achieve. Your future depends not only on your ability but on your mind-set.

—KENNETH L. OTTO, senior vice-president
Tenneco, Inc.

In the American lexicon, "life-style" has become one of those catchall words used to describe the way individuals, groups, or even nations typically go about their daily living. Medically, we talk about a positive or negative life-style's influence on health. In my experience many busy executives focus attention on long-term health and fitness issues, but often neglect simple daily living practices that have a profound influence on their health, performance, and overall happiness.

Like it or not, your daily life-style does have an impact on your health. In an important series of papers in the 1970s, researchers in California surveying 7,000 adults found seven personal practices that highly correlate with physical health:

1. Sleeping seven or eight hours a night
2. Eating breakfast almost every day
3. Never or rarely eating between meals

122

4. Being at or near prescribed height-adjusted weight
5. Never smoking cigarettes
6. Moderate or no use of alcohol
7. Regular physical activity

Individuals who followed most or all of these practices were found to have better health than those who didn't. More important, in a five-year follow-up, those who followed these practices had a significantly lower mortality rate than those who did not.

If your body were a machine, these seven regular personal health practices would all be part of the preventive maintenance needed to keep it running smoothly. It's more than just being healthy; it's living to *stay* healthy. An extremely important part of health maintenance is regular physical checkups, in which you work with your doctor to stay fit (more on this later in this chapter). Another is the concept of risk factor reduction. A risk factor is any condition or practice that predisposes you to, or increases your likelihood of, developing a disease. Some risk factors are at least partially genetic (for example, family history of coronary heart disease [CHD], diabetes); others relate to daily habits that are under your control, such as cigarette smoking, alcohol consumption, and a sedentary life-style.

SMOKING

No topic aroused more adamant reactions during our executive interviews than smoking. Not smoking was cited in our survey as the most "extremely important" factor in maintaining good health, ahead of both regular exercise and proper diet. Here, as in other fitness-related areas, there has been a dramatic change among executives. Some 56% of our survey respondents at some time smoked cigarettes. Only 10% remain smokers. Indeed, most of the executives reported that the reduction of cigarette smoking in corporate offices is one of the most striking trends they have witnessed in the past 10 years. "It used to be when you went to a meeting, say in the boardroom with twenty people, you'd find well over half of them smoking," noted Navistar's Donald Lennox. "Now it's rare to have anybody light up a cigarette."

Before we become too self-congratulatory about declining cigarette smoking among executives, however, several important issues should be addressed. First, a major health problem still exists. The fact that 1 in 10 of the top executives in our survey still exposes himself to the health risks of smoking is still far too high. Cigarette smoking is the major factor in more than 350,000 deaths annually in the United States. It is estimated that it accounts for almost one-third of all heart disease and cancer deaths. (Although pipe and cigar smoking are less associated with CHD and lung cancer, they carry virtually the same risk as cigarette smoking for cancers of the larynx and oral cavity.) If you smoke from one to two packs of cigarettes a day, you decrease your life expectancy by at least five—and perhaps over eight—years. At the two-pack range, you lose an average of 5½ minutes of life every time you light up.

In short, giving up cigarettes is a powerful positive health decision. The risk of developing CHD due to smoking drops 50% by one year after stopping; after five years, former smokers have less than half the chance of developing lung cancer than those who smoke.

Second, smokers pose important health risks for those around them, including family as well as coworkers. Nonsmokers who inhale smoke from a nearby cigarette ("sidestream" smoke) or smoke exhaled by a smoker ("mainstream" smoke) are called passive smokers because their exposure comes from merely being in the presence of someone who smokes. Passive smoking increases the likelihood of allergic attacks, respiratory infections, and the onset of angina in individuals with CHD.

With the overwhelming evidence of the health risks of smoking, it is hard to believe that any informed adult, particularly one in an executive position who is used to making decisions based on an objective evaluation of data, still smokes. The answer to this paradox undoubtedly lies in the powerful addicting quality of cigarette smoking. As one CEO who still smokes lamented: "I'm addicted. I got addicted when I was very young. It was considered a rite of passage from boyhood to manhood to start smoking; it was a very popular thing to do. I have stopped periodically, but I'm not fooling myself. I know it's going to cut some years off my life. . . . When I see kids smoking—my children do not smoke—I feel like grabbing them and saying, 'Don't do that or you will be fighting it for the rest of your life, as I have.' "

Indeed, it is thought that nicotine can be as addictive as heroin. The National Institute of Mental Health has established a new classification of mental illness called "Tobacco Dependence Disorder" for individuals who are unable to stop smoking despite awareness of the medical consequences.

Still, millions of Americans and 698 out of our survey sample of 1,139 top executives have stopped smoking. How? Although formal smoking cessation programs have been effective for many, the majority of the population at large and all of the executives we interviewed who have stopped smoking have done so without such programs. In one way or another, they finally accepted the fact that they were only hurting themselves. "You know that the lung cancer risks are great and that lung cancer is a fatal disease. Yet somehow it's hard to relate those consequences to your own cigarette smoking," explained Lin Patterson, president and CEO of Appleton & Lange. "So the way I stopped smoking was to shrink my self-interest. I kept thinking, 'This is unhealthy. Why am I doing this to my body?' I was determined to stop and eventually got the thought that it was an unhealthy thing to do firmly planted in my mind."

Nationally, the single most effective incentive for giving up smoking is the occurrence of an individual's first heart attack. Even a scare will often do it. Here's how one *Fortune* 500 CEO had his "self-interest" brought forcibly home to him: "I had gone in for a company physical, and I had a heart stress test that showed an abnormality. So I had an angiogram, which was normal and showed that the stress test had been a false positive. I was very fortunate. But the whole process scared me enough so that I crumbled up the cigarettes and threw them away."

Smoking for top executives, like being overweight, can pose detrimental image problems as well as health problems. And, as is often the case, some of smoking's severest judges are ex-smokers. Observed Donald Lennox, who kicked a two-pack-a-day habit: "Once the body of knowledge had grown to the point where it was clear that cigarette smoking was detrimental to my health and not worth it, I said, 'I'm gonna quit.' And I did. I just can't understand and get very frustrated with people who say, 'I wish I could quit smoking.' For Christ's sake, just quit them. You have to wonder if there is a relationship between the ability to run a major corporation and the ability to have the self-discipline it takes to do these things."

CANCER

Cancer is the second leading cause of death in the United States. In 1987, it is estimated that almost 500,000 people died from some form of cancer.

In contrast to heart disease, for which there is at least some recognition that daily life-style habits can play a role, there continues to be considerable free-floating anxiety and much less concrete positive action concerning cancer. It is a very poorly understood problem in both the general and executive populations.

The major hurdle that must be overcome is the prevalent perception that cancer is an act of God, unrelated to personal habits and choices. A national poll conducted in 1984 found that 46% of adult Americans believe "there is not much a person can do about cancer" and almost half did not identify cancer as a disease that could be influenced by people's life-styles. This is particularly distressing since it is now estimated that between 70% and 80% of all cancers could be prevented with careful attention to daily habits and practices.

The risks of cigarette smoking have already been stated; it is estimated that eliminating cigarettes would eliminate 35% of cancers. Poor nutrition and dietary habits may play a role in up to 30% of malignancies. Obesity increases the likelihood of colon, breast, and uterine cancers. Virtually all of the nonmelanoma forms of skin cancer detected each year are related to excessive exposure to the sun. Heavy alcohol consumption is associated with cancers of the liver, esophagus, throat, and larynx. In all of these situations, minimal changes in daily life-style habits can significantly decrease your risk of cancer.

The individual also plays a key role in the early detection of cancer. Regular self-examination for signs of cancer is extremely important in addition to cancer surveillance as part of every routine physical examination. This is an area where your physician can help you.

In a number of studies, more than 40% of patients who detected signs or symptoms suggestive of cancer delayed seeking a diagnosis for more than three months. Such delays have a markedly adverse effect on the likelihood of survival. The warning signs of cancer should be approached with the same decisive action applied to business problems.

There is great interest among those in the medical community in several recent studies that have linked active life-styles with a decreased risk of some kinds of cancer. In one study, athletic women were found to have a lower risk of breast and reproductive system cancers than nonathletic women. Other studies have found a higher incidence of colon cancers in sedentary individuals than more active individuals, although this may be partially explained by the fact that people who exercise have more regular bowel movements.

While definitive links between exercise and cancer reduction have not yet been established, we are at a point where we can list regular exercise as a preventive life-style measure that can be taken to lower the risk of cancer. This is precisely what the American Cancer Society did in its recent booklet, *Taking Charge*.

GENETIC RISK FACTORS

Two risk factors are not under an individual's control—that is, they can't be avoided by changes in daily habits—a family history of CHD and diabetes. If you have either of these risk factors, you should monitor your health very closely to keep other risk factors low. Too often, executives and their physicians take the risk factors associated with family illnesses too lightly. Let me give you an example. We know that a family history of premature CHD (blood relatives who have had symptomatic coronary disease prior to age 65) predisposes an individual to developing the same problem. Not long ago, I had dinner with a young executive who mentioned that his father had suffered a heart attack at the age of 35 and that several uncles had undergone coronary artery bypass surgery in their forties. He was 42 and had just been appointed president of a division of his company. His physician had advised him that as long as he was not having any symptoms not to worry.

This attitude was much too cavalier. At the very minimum, this young executive should have a detailed knowledge of his cholesterol, be on a regular exercise program, avoid cigarette smoking (he already was), and have a yearly physical examination with special attention to the cardiovascular system, including blood pressure determination, cardiac examination, and electrocardiogram. He couldn't do anything to change his family history of CHD, but he needed to pay special attention to keeping his other risk factors low.

Similarly, diabetics should be under close medical supervision and pay scrupulous attention to controlling their condition and reducing other risk factors. Diabetics are twice as likely to develop CHD, twice as likely to suffer a stroke, and five times as likely to develop arterial disease of the extremities as nondiabetics.

The risk factor of diabetes also interacts synergistically with other risk factors. A diabetic who also smokes cigarettes and has high blood pressure and elevated blood cholesterol has 12 times the risk of developing CHD than an individual without diabetes who has no risk factors.

Diabetes is a complicated, often hereditary, disorder of carbohydrate metabolism that affects between 4% and 6% of the adult population in the United States. The incidence of diabetes in our executive survey mirrored this statistic, with 3% of respondents reporting this condition.

There are two major types of diabetes. Type I (also called insulin-dependent diabetes) typically occurs in young people, often with onset in teenage years, and requires insulin to control glucose levels. This type of diabetes represents about 10% of cases. Type II diabetes (also called non-insulin-dependent diabetes), representing the other 90% of cases, typically has its onset in the middle years (fifties and sixties) and typically does not require insulin for control. Oral medication and strict dietary control of glucose are usually sufficient treatment.

Since the cause of diabetes is unknown, reducing the risk factor per se is not possible. It is important to control associated and exacerbating conditions, however, in order to keep overall risk factors under good control. Obesity aggravates diabetes, so ideal weight should be maintained. Diabetics should follow diets low in cholesterol and saturated fats, avoid cigarettes, and keep blood pressure under good control.

HEALTH EVALUATION

Many executives used to resist undergoing physical examinations, espousing the philosophy "if it ain't broke, don't fix it." Yet in the past 10 to 20 years there has been increasingly widespread acceptance of the wisdom of regular checkups as a key part of preventive maintenance—a positive step in remaining healthy and fit. In fact, periodic examinations have become deeply ingrained in the personal health maintenance programs of top executives and the corporate health programs of most major companies.

In our survey of top executives whose average age was slightly more than 50, 81% had undergone a complete physical exam in the previous two years, with 57% having had one within the past year. (The leaders here were *Fortune* 500 executives, 77% of whom had had a complete exam within the past year.) Fully 99% of the respondents had had a physical within the previous four years.

In the absence of specific medical problems, I typically recommend that individuals over the age of 30 visit a physician on a yearly basis. As will be subsequently discussed in detail, for individuals between the ages of 30 and 49, not all of these visits will be for comprehensive evaluations. I recommend comprehensive physical examinations every three years for executives between the ages of 30 and 39, every two years between the ages of 40 and 49, and every year from the age of 50 and older. While there is some debate about the need for a yearly physician visit below age 50, I strongly advocate one. This enables you and your physician to monitor your ongoing health status (weight, blood pressure, cholesterol, and so on) and to discuss other health and fitness issues, such as your exercise routine, and any problems or injuries that might have occurred.

Another source of controversy surrounding physical examinations or "health evaluations," as they are more properly called, is what they should consist of. A number of national task forces have issued guidelines on what they perceive to be justified and valuable components of a physical examination for adults of various ages. The American Cancer Society, Mayo Clinic, Cleveland Clinic, our own Center for Health and Fitness at the University of Massachusetts Medical School, and other health care institutions have also developed guidelines on this topic.

Based on this extensive literature, knowledge of the unique pressures and concerns of executives, and my own clinical practice, the guidelines for periodic health and fitness evaluations for busy executives listed in this chapter are reasonable. Every patient has his or her own distinct physical, psychological, and emotional makeup. There are thus no perfect guidelines for every situation.

What this book should help you avoid, however, is the cursory visit to your physician's office where you're told that "you look just great" but learn nothing about how you're actually doing and the kind of issues you should be concerned about to preserve your health and reduce risks. In-depth counseling and fitness prescription should be included in every complete physical examination. Equally important, I want to help you avoid excessive tests, in the absence of clear-cut indications, that may expose you to certain risks, such as the radiation involved in GI series tests.

A final note: Your comprehensive examination will not be "comprehensive" unless you have established a relationship with a physician who is knowledgeable about exercise, nutrition, and risk factor reduction, as well as more traditional health matters. In the past, few doctors viewed their role as going beyond the basics. Today they are much more aware of the need to treat the whole person. It is reasonable for you to expect your physician to give you sound, practical advice on all facets of your daily personal health habits.

129

EARLY YEARS

While most youngsters have annual checkups as part of their regular medical care (or as required by school, camp, and so on), the first adult examination should occur at about age 18. Although this does not directly involve executives, many have teenage children and inquire about when and if their offspring should be evaluated. Eighteen is the age when many teenagers leave home for the first extended period, either to attend college or get a job. It's a good time to check their blood pressure and cholesterol level and to provide counseling on exercise, nutrition, alcohol consumption, and safety habits. In the current climate, it's also a critical opportunity to provide information on sexual habits and AIDS.

Ideally, another general examination should be done in a person's mid-twenties, when he or she leaves college or graduate school to settle into a job and life-style with different pressures and concerns. Many epidemiologists argue that the period right after college graduation is the key time to interact with young adults concerning life-style and health. Exercise programs, in particular, are often in jeopardy when the young adult makes the transition from the convenience and atmosphere of college athletic facilities. Weight, blood pressure, and cholesterol level should be obtained once again, and appropriate counseling on weight control, nutrition, and exercise offered.

Such early health evaluations also offer the opportunity to look for any high school- or college-related athletic injuries and correct them before they become chronic adult problems. Among adults in their forties, for example, many of the knee injuries being attributed to running can be traced back to high school and college basketball or football injuries left untreated during the individual's twenties and thirties. Many of these chronically injured knees are fine to walk around on but become very sore when the 40-year-old decides to start a jogging program.

GENERAL GUIDELINES FOR EXAMINATIONS

As stated earlier, in the absence of specific medical problems or symptoms, I recommend a complete physical examination every year for executives starting at the age of 50; every other year for those age 40 to 49; and every third year for those age 30 to 39. The complete exam should include all the elements of a routine office checkup, plus a series of laboratory tests and cardiovascular fitness, body fat, and musculoskeletal tests. It should also include self-examination advice, counseling, and fitness prescription.

Executives between the ages of 39 and 49 should have an annual checkup in the years between their comprehensive evaluations. The examination protocol is a streamlined version of the comprehensive physical. Weight, blood pressure, and cholesterol level should be checked, as well as general musculoskeletal condition and any signs of cancer. In addition, exercise prescription should be evaluated and updated. This visit also provides a valuable opportunity to discuss any problems that have arisen since the previous comprehensive evaluation.

The table on page 140 summarizes my guidelines for the physical evaluation and, according to age, the frequency (in years) in which they should be performed. These are outlined in more depth below. But first, let's address two other concerns: your dental health and your visual health. One CEO I interviewed had just returned from a painful dental appointment for root canal work and complained that taking care of his teeth was "a continual losing battle." Unfortunately, this nihilistic attitude is not uncommon among busy executives.

It doesn't have to be this way. Your teeth should last a lifetime, and with proper preventive care you can avoid a lot of the misery of tooth decay and gum disease. Unfortunately, this message hasn't reached enough of the adult population. Only 50% of the population visits a dentist on a yearly basis (still not often enough—every six months is preferable). Only 65% brush their teeth at least once a day and only 38% use dental floss regularly. Given these statistics, it's no surprise that 75% of the adult population develops periodontal (gum) disease.

Why bother? Aside from the obvious issue of avoiding the pain and cost of major dental work, healthy teeth are essential for good appearance and proper nutrition. Poor teeth also contribute to systemic illnesses such as infections. A reasonable program for avoiding gum and tooth disease includes twice-a-day brushing and flossing and twice-a-year preventive visits to a dentist throughout adult life.

For executives, in particular, who spend a great deal of time reading, visual health is just as important. There is a tendency among executives to put off going to an eye doctor even when they notice they are having problems—after all, they reason, they can see "OK." Don't! Serious eye problems can develop, particularly as you get older. In the absence of any symptoms, I recommend a visit to an ophthalmologist every five years between the ages of 30 and 49 and every three to four years over age 50. Tonometry (a test for glaucoma) should be performed in your early fifties and then every five years thereafter.

One topic not included among the physical examination guidelines but that nonetheless is important for you and your physician to assess periodically is your immunization status. It is often forgotten. Tetanus and diphtheria immunizations should be brought up to date every 10 years. The completeness of the immunization program received as a child should be assessed at some point during an adult's early thirties. For executives who travel internationally, the specific immunization status for various geographic areas where travel is planned should be assessed periodically.

In addition, executives over age 50 should have an annual flu shot. In some instances, executives over 60 or those with significant underlying symptoms should also have pneumovax, a vaccine that protects against certain kinds of pneumonia. Check with your physician to find out if this latter recommendation applies to you.

Here are specific recommendations of various evaluations and prescriptions, by age category, for executive health maintenance.

GENERAL GUIDELINES/PHYSICAL EXAMINATION

Age 30 to 39

Special emphasis should be placed on weight, blood pressure, and cardiac exam. The arms and legs should also be carefully examined for any signs of joint injury, loss of flexibility, or muscle weakness. A cancer checkup should be part of the physical examination. For all individuals this includes complete examination of the skin (with the individual disrobed), thyroid, lymph nodes, and oral cavity. In addition, for men, examination of the testicles, prostate, and rectum should be performed. For women, a breast exam and pelvic exam with pap smear should be performed.

Age 40 to 49

All of the evaluations and cancer screening outlined above (age 30 to 39) should be performed for 40- to 49-year-old executives as well. In addition, visual acuity should be formally tested at least once between age 40 and 50. A digital rectal examination should be performed on a yearly basis over age 40 to rule out colon cancer, and a stool sample should be checked for occult blood (blood in stools which is not visible except through your doctor's test).

Age 50 and older

The same general framework for a complete physical examination should be followed as outlined for executives between the ages of 30 and 49. However, since the incidence of both CHD and various types of cancer becomes appreciably greater by the fifties, the search for early detection of these problems—either by history or physical exam findings—becomes extremely important.

All of the evaluations outlined for 30- to 49-year-old executives should be performed on individuals age 50 and older. In addition, an evaluation of the rectum by sigmoidoscopy (a procedure in which a clear plastic tube is inserted in the rectum to look for visual signs of cancer) should be performed twice—a year apart—in the early fifties to rule out rectal cancer. If these two evaluations are normal, the procedure can then be repeated every three to five years. Stools should be checked yearly for the presence of occult blood. Women over 50 should have yearly mammography in addition to a manual breast exam and pelvic exam with pap smear.

In addition to visual acuity tests every three to five years, hearing tests should also be performed several times during the fifties and then every three to five years thereafter. Tonometry (a test for glaucoma) should also be performed in the early fifties and then every five years after that.

LABORATORY TESTS

Age 30 to 39

Cholesterol level and blood sugar should be obtained every three years during this decade. A hematocrit and other blood chemistries are required only if symptoms are present or you are at high risk for a problem. For example, kidney function tests (BUN, creatinine) are advisable for individuals with high blood pressure, liver function tests for those who consume large amounts of alcohol, and hematocrit for individuals who complain of fatigue. Urine should be analyzed for protein, blood, and cells every three years.

Electrocardiograms should also be obtained every three years, (these undoubtedly will be required for company insurance policies anyway). In addition, women between the ages of 35 and 40 should have a baseline mammography performed every three years.

Age 40 to 49

All of the laboratory tests outlined for 30- to 39-year-olds should be obtained; however, the frequency should be increased from once every three years to once every two years. A test of cholesterol level and a resting electrocardiogram should be performed annually for 40- to 49-year-old executives.

Age 50 and older

All of the laboratory tests outlined for 30- to 49-year-olds should also be performed on executives age 50 and older on a yearly basis. Yearly cholesterol measurements and resting electrocardiograms are particularly important.

ASSESSMENT OF CARDIOVASCULAR FITNESS

Age 30 to 39

A formal exercise tolerance test (ETT) with full monitoring on a treadmill is not required in this age group in the absence of risk factors or symptoms. It is advisable, however, to obtain an ETT every three years if you smoke or have high blood pressure or high cholesterol. For individuals under age 40, the assessment of cardiovascular fitness should be performed by an exercise physiologist who can evaluate heart rate response to exercise exertion and develop an aerobic exercise prescription.

Age 40 to 49

During the decade between 40 and 50 the formal evaluation of cardiovascular fitness should be performed every other year using the techniques outlined for 30- to 39-year-old executives. There is one important change, however, which involves the use of a fully monitored, graded ETT. If the individual has no risk factors or symptoms of CHD, the ETT should not be used as a screening test to try to pick up occult CHD. However, individuals over 45 who have previously been inactive and wish to start an exercise program should undergo a fully monitored ETT prior to starting their program. In addition, inactive individuals over 40 who have any risk factors for CHD and intend to start a new exercise program should also have an ETT prior to beginning a program.

Age 50 and older

Most of the considerations outlined for 40- to 49-year-olds are also relevant to executives over 50. Several issues merit particular attention, however. First, by the time a male executive reaches age 55, he has a 33% chance of having CHD and by age 60, there is a 20% chance that he will have already suffered a heart attack. This doesn't mean that cardiovascular fitness is irrelevant—far from it. Individuals with CHD or those recovering from a heart attack stand to benefit as much or more from improved cardiovascular fitness as do individuals without heart problems. It simply means that more caution must be exercised in assessing cardiovascular fitness and a more thorough evaluation must be undertaken for early symptoms of CHD.

As described for executives aged 30 to 49, a monitored ETT should not be undertaken as a screening procedure in an asymptomatic individual over age 50 who has no risk factors for CHD. However, all individuals over 50 who have been previously inactive and wish to start a new exercise program should have a fully monitored, maximum ETT under medical supervision prior to starting the program.

BODY FAT

Age 30 to 39

Percentage of body fat is best measured by using the skin fold caliper technique or by underwater weighing (the latter procedure requires the specialized facilities of a major center). These are much more accurate than simple weighing in determining what percentage of an individual's weight is fat. A body-fat assessment should be conducted every three years.

Age 40 to 49

Assessment of body fat either by the skinfold caliper technique or underwater weighing should be performed every two years.

Age 50 and older

Annual determination of body fat for executives over age 50 is worthwhile. Since there is much more experience with the skin fold caliper technique than the underwater weighing technique in this age range, it is the preferred method.

MUSCULOSKELETAL EXAMINATION

Age 30 to 39

Here the strength and flexibility of muscles are assessed and joints inspected for any signs of prior injury. Such an evaluation requires some specialized equipment and takes about 30 minutes. Performed by a physical therapist, it is important for both injury assessment and prevention. Most private physicians do not have the equipment to conduct this comprehensive exam, but should still do a somewhat more limited assessment as part of the comprehensive physical examination every three years.

Age 40 to 49

The comprehensive musculoskeletal evaluation outlined for 30- to 39-year-old executives should also be performed for 40- to 49-year-olds. The frequency should be increased from every three to every two years.

Age 50 and older

A similar protocol as that outlined for individuals 30 to 49 should be followed. Increased attention should be paid to examining joints for any early signs of arthritis. The examination should be performed on a yearly basis.

SELF-EXAMINATION

Age 30 to 39

Unfortunately, this important part of the health evaluation is often neglected. The individual should be taught either testicular or breast self-examination and skin self-examination. Since testicular or breast cancers are significant causes of death in men and women of this age, you should perform the appropriate exam on yourself monthly. Your physician can show you how.

Age 40 to 49

Monthly self-examinations of the skin and testicles or breasts remain important during your forties.

Age 50 and older

Knowing how to conduct monthly skin and testicular or breast exams becomes increasingly important in this age range. At age 50 and beyond, however, it is particularly important to have detailed discussions about what do and do not constitute worrisome symptoms. You should discuss with your physician, for example, any change in bowel habits, any evidence of blood in the stools, or any worrisome chest symptoms.

FITNESS PRESCRIPTIONS

Age 30 to 39

In the decade between 30 and 39, discuss both aerobic exercise and musculoskeletal exercise with your doctor and set up a specific plan. In our medical center, for example, such an initial discussion is held with a physician, followed by a 30-minute session with an exercise specialist during which techniques for aerobic conditioning and strength and flexibility training are demonstrated and specific questions are answered. Excellent sources of exercise prescriptions are available to you and your physician (such as those offered in chapter 3). The advice to "go out and get a little more exercise" is no longer state-of-the-art. You should leave your comprehensive health evaluation with a specific exercise program that can be initiated the next day.

Age 40 to 49

Like executives in their thirties, those between ages 40 and 49 should be given specific exercise guidelines for a program they can carry out on a regular basis. Again, it is important to have the kind of ongoing relationship with your physician that allows your exercise program to satisfy health and fitness needs as well as blend into a realistic view of your aspirations and life-style. Adopting fitness programs that can be shared with other family members also becomes an increasingly relevant issue for 40- to 49-year-old executives.

Your exercise prescription should have aerobic exercise at its core and also include some exercises to build musculoskeletal endurance and maintain or enhance flexibility. Any preexisting conditions, such as knee or back problems, as well as the types of activity you enjoy, should be factored in. Your physician, perhaps working with an exercise physiologist, should be able to give you specific guidance on the right program for you (such as those offered in chapter 3).

Age 50 and older

Knowledge of the physiology of exercise in individuals over age 50 has exploded in the past five years. Several important studies have shown that age-related declines in cardiovascular endurance and strength can be dramatically reduced by properly designed, consistent exercise programs. In some instances, substantial *improvements* in cardiovascular endurance have been achieved even in populations where they were not expected.

For example, in our Exercise Physiology Laboratory at the University of Massachusetts Medical School, we studied a group of healthy individuals between ages 70 and 79 (average: 74) enrolled in a 12-week supervised walking regimen. At the end of the study, the average cardiovascular endurance had improved by 12%—a gain comparable to what you would expect if you started previously inactive 20- or 30-year-olds on a new exercise program.

Issues of safety in exercise prescription are particularly important for individuals over 50. For this reason, such programs should be initiated under medical guidance—preferably at a center with background and expertise in this area.

COUNSELING

Age 30 to 39

Counseling sessions with your physician are a particularly important part of both the comprehensive health evaluations that should take place every three years in this age group and the streamlined office visits that should be made annually. Such sessions provide an excellent opportunity for you and your doctor to discuss your overall health and fitness status and the directions you should be taking in the next year to reduce risk factors and optimize your health. The issues of weight, nutrition, alcohol, cardiac risk factors, exercise, stress, and life-style should all be included in these discussions.

Age 40 to 49

Establishing an ongoing relationship with a physician pays dividends at any age but assumes increasing importance as you enter your forties. By this time, many executives have reached positions of considerable authority. In addition, most have also taken on important family obligations. Not only are the responsibilities and pressures greater, but the health risks for such problems as CHD and cancer also increase.

While episodic care with a physician who does not know you is never a good way to manage your health, it becomes even worse by the time you are in your forties. Many health-related decisions are not black-and-white but come in many shades of gray. The best decisions on a variety of health and fitness issues come out of an ongoing relationship between you and your physician.

The issues of risk factor reduction, nutrition, stress, and exercise should be discussed in detail during your visits for health evaluations, and these are best done with a physician who knows your medical history and goals, pressures, and aspirations.

Age 50 and older

The decade between 50 and 60 is a watershed for most executives. By their mid-fifties, most have reached as high as they are going to rise in major corporations and both business and personal issues take on a different aura. The challenges of maintaining pace and vigor begin to loom larger.

Counseling executives over the age of 50 represents at once an extremely worthwhile, challenging, and delicate task for a physician. On the one hand, there are a number of important health issues to discuss; on the other hand, the physician is often dealing with very senior managers who know their own minds and are used to soliciting a variety of opinions prior to making any important decision. Dr. Edward J. Bernacki, who has had many years' experience handling such matters,

GUIDELINES FOR EXECUTIVE HEALTH EVALUATION

Factor	Age/Frequency (years)		
	30–39	40–49	50+
Physical Exam			
Weight	1	1	1
Blood pressure	1	1	1
Cardiac exam	1	1	1
Limbs (muscles, joints)	1	1	1
Thyroid, lymph, oral cavity	1	1	1
Testicles, prostate, rectal (men)	1	1	1
Breast, pelvic/pap (women)	1	1	1
Lab tests			
Digital rectal exam	—	1	1
Sigmoidoscopy/stool check	—	—	1/3–5*
Cholesterol level	3	1	1
Electrocardiogram	3	1	1
Blood sugar**	3	2	1
Urine	3	2	1
Mammography (women)	3†	2	1
Other Tests			
Cardiovascular fitness	3	2	1
Body fat	3	2	1
Musculoskeletal‡	3	2	1

Source: Compiled by the author.

*Yearly basis twice in early fifties; if normal, repeat every three to five years.

**Other blood tests may be required if symptoms are present or an individual is at high risk for a problem.

†Mammographies should be performed in women over 35 years old.

‡This requires specialized equipment that your physician may not have. If symptoms are present, the exam can be performed by a physical therapist at a specialized facility.

first as senior physician at United Technologies and then as vice-president of health, environmental medicine, and safety at Tenneco, describes how he handles executive health:

> Many senior executives approach their health in the same way they would approach a business decision . . . often they're not going to take advice. They're going to talk about it, analyze it, get fifteen opinions . . . so in essence, I plant the thought. I don't get too excited if my initial recommendations are kind of put on the shelf so they can think about others. Eventually they'll do the right thing if you handle them gently.

Key matters to be discussed in annual sessions include, of course, any symptoms that are worrying you, as well as nutrition, risk factor reduction, and exercise. In the past 10 years, medical research has demonstrated that reducing the risk of CHD and cancer in individuals over age 50 is just as relevant as for younger executives. A trusting relationship with a physician can even foster discussions of a variety of personal issues and fears concerning slowing down and retirement. It's important to remember that an individual who reaches the age of 65 in our society has an 80% chance of reaching the age of 80. Long-term planning is not irrelevant.

It is very clear that much of what we used to feel were physiologic age-related declines in cardiovascular endurance and muscular strength are related to decreased activity rather than aging per se. Yet, after age 50 some of the safety issues related to exercise become highly relevant. The annual comprehensive health evaluation becomes a key time to focus on these issues.

7

Setting Up a Corporate Program

I'd hate to offer a program for 10,000 people on the basis of "you do this—it's going to save the company money." That makes no sense; it's not important that the wellness center save the company money. What is important is that the wellness center saves lives and makes people's lives better and happier. The spin-off, by God, is a person who's going to work harder for you. He's going to be happy at work. He's going to be more productive, more creative. And, he's going to be there more often.

—WILLIAM COORS, chairman
Adolph Coors Company

This is a book about personal health and fitness for executives. It focuses on the personal decisions executives make on a daily basis and the habits they adopt that either enhance or detract from their health, fitness, and performance. Yet, there is another important area in which the decisions of top executives have an impact on health and fitness, and it involves their employees. What are companies doing to ensure the "wellness" of their work forces?

During the past five years, our researchers have visited and talked with people from corporate fitness programs at AT&T, Coors, IBM, Johnson & Johnson, Kimberly-Clark, PepsiCo, Sentry Insurance, Tenneco, and many others. We've also talked to many entrepreneurs managing smaller companies about what they realistically can—and cannot—hope to accomplish in providing health and fitness opportunities for their employees. The purpose of this chapter is to examine ways that companies can exert a positive impact on the health and fitness of their employees and to offer a prescription for a healthy corporate America.

Executive opinions about corporate fitness programs vary widely. Some CEOs, such as William Coors of Adolph Coors and J. L. Ketelsen of Tenneco, are staunch advocates of company-sponsored employee fitness programs. Others feel equally strongly that health and fitness matters involve personal decisions and the company should stay out of them. Many executives in smaller companies, despite their desire to launch such programs, encounter the additional problem of limited financial resources. "It's about the last thing a banker or investor wants to hear about," lamented one entrepreneur.

Based on the current levels of interest and debate, how companies should relate to the health and fitness of their employees promises to be one of the major corporate issues of the 1990s. The number of firms that have already established formal fitness programs is staggering. An estimated 50,000 companies have programs in place and more than 400 have hired full-time fitness directors. The overall issue of how to facilitate employee health is even more pervasive. I could not find a single top executive who had not given this matter considerable thought. It is clear that these executives are concerned not only about their own health and fitness but also about the health of their employees.

In part, the interest in employee health is based on economic considerations. In many corporations health and insurance benefits are one of the major expenses, and in some instances they are the major expense. In an article titled "How Companies Tackle Health Care Costs," published by the *Harvard Business Review* in 1985, Warren Loomis, president of Dexter Corp., is quoted as saying:

> Health benefits are now the third largest cost element after raw materials and straight time pay for most manufacturers, second for most service businesses. Any president who isn't giving the control of health benefits significant attention doesn't yet understand the magnitude of the problem.

Most companies have tackled the health care cost problem with such strategies as copayments and other financing packages that provide employees with the incentive to use health care efficiently. In addition, corporate fitness and wellness programs have been proposed as a means of ultimately reducing the high costs of certain chronic diseases where life-style (for example, cigarette smoking, obesity, and inactivity) place employees at higher risk.

The issue of whether corporate fitness programs save the company money has been hotly debated. In reviews of corporate programs conducted by the Washington Business Group on Health and Arthur D. Little, it was concluded that long-term savings of between $3 and $6 could be expected for every $1 spent. Several in-house studies, including those conducted by Tenneco and the Canadian Life Assurance Co., show that participants in corporate fitness programs cost the corporation less in health care expenditures than did nonparticipants. In Tenneco's case, however, there were also differences prior to initiation of the program (exercisers cost less in terms of health care dollars before a corporate fitness program was started).

Most executives agree with William Coors that the main motivation for establishing a program is not to save the company money but to do something positive for employees and to improve morale. This is consistent with data from several major surveys showing that more than twice as many executives support corporate fitness as a morale booster than as a cost-containment measure.

Plans that help employees take charge of their lives and health will ultimately save companies health care dollars. Yet, the best way to weigh such plans is in the context suggested by William Coors and his counterparts—namely that health and fitness programs should be offered as a gesture of caring for the employees, with the expectation that healthier, more fit workers will also be more productive. In short, health, fitness, and performance are strongly linked.

Several aspects of the cost effectiveness debate are frequently overlooked, including those that relate to the issues of turnover, absenteeism, and recruitment. Data from the Tenneco fitness program show that participants are less likely to be absent and less likely to leave the company than nonparticipants. "There's no question that participation in the [corporate fitness] program reduces turnover, and turnover is expensive," commented Tenneco chairman and CEO J. L. Ketelsen. "We learned that people who participate are more likely to stay with the company."

While reduced absenteeism and turnover are decided benefits, the most important gain achieved by companies that have established fitness facilities is improved morale. "The program has succeeded beyond my wildest dreams," said Ketelsen, whose company built a fully equipped fitness center. "We've had much more participation than we ever expected. When we built the center everybody said, 'Well, it'll get old and usage will decline.' But it hasn't; in fact, the percentages are going up. . . . I think it's the best thing we've ever done for our people. We could have given them raises equal to the cost of the facility and it wouldn't have made nearly the same impact."

Improved employee morale is based on the fact that corporate fitness facilities provide a symbol of how companies feel about their employees. "It's an employer's responsibility to be concerned about the health and well-being of his people. And it should be perceived by the employees as just that—concern," stressed William Coors. "If we can develop an atmosphere of concern and trust, where our people have faith that we have their best interests at heart and that we're going to use our resources to determine the best and most effective treatments, then they will give us *their* best."

How a corporate fitness program is structured can also make a powerful statement about how a company's executives view its employees and the world. "We viewed fitness as something that more and more people were interested in, and we strongly wanted to do something that was for all employees from top to bottom, from the chairman to the maintenance staff," explained Tenneco's Kenneth L. Otto. "The fitness center accomplished a number of things, not the least of which is that it helped employees recognize that we are a people-oriented company."

One by-product of the Tenneco facility that surprised senior managers is the degree to which the common exercise center enhanced communication. "I've learned more about this company in the shower room and locker room—meeting, running, and exercising with people that I never would have met before," Otto observed. "I can personally stop more stupid rumors at that level. I can say to people, 'You go out and tell everybody that is wrong—Otto says so.' "

When all the attributes of a facility such as Tenneco's are taken together—the morale, communication, caring for the employee, and egalitarian spirit—they begin to describe what many people have called the "culture" of a company. Much has been written on corporate culture, and most top executives think long and hard about how to build a positive culture within their companies. In many instances a fitness center serves as a focal point of company pride and symbolizes what the company is all about.

A senior vice-president of Chase Manhattan Bank noted that no recruit being considered for a job leaves the bank without seeing its fitness facility. "We're in competition with all the other major financial institutions in New York," he said. "The fitness center says a lot about Chase Manhattan and gives us a significant edge with the best and brightest young people coming out in financial services."

A number of CEOs emphasized that their fitness and athletic programs are central to their corporate cultures. "Playing sports together affects how you feel about the company," said John Bierwirth. "It's not necessarily athletics that gives the company a winning attitude, but it can be that. It certainly can be a sense of being on a team together, and God knows that's been important at Grumman. . . . I think our people know each other as human beings."

Robert Rechholtz links the fitness program at Coors to a corporate philosophy that places a premium on quality for both its people and products. When asked to describe how Coors's fitness program relates to its corporate culture, he replied: "We strive for quality in all we are and do. . . . Coors has a strong corporate plan and culture. I've worked for three number-one corporations: Procter & Gamble, RJ Reynolds, and Gallo. All have one thing in common: keen awareness of the importance of product quality and a discipline to pursue it . . . but none of them has the simple, credible dedication to quality in products, people, and working atmosphere that Coors has. William Coors has worked to make it a high priority. . . . [For example,] in the wellness program, a lot of people use it and the fun, competition, and involvement are incredible. Even some people who initially scoffed at the program now are enthusiastic members."

An issue directly related to corporate culture is the image the company presents to the outside world. Many companies spend millions of dollars annually trying to create an identity and "position." Executives in many of the companies that have made a major commitment to corporate fitness credit their programs for making a tremendous contribution to how the world at large views their company.

Dr. Dennis Colacino, who played a major role in organizing the PepsiCo corporate fitness program, told me that Donald Kennedy, the chairman of PepsiCo, intended the program to help senior management look and feel like the theme from the company's advertising: "Comin' at ya, goin' strong." Robert Rechholtz at Coors related how the company's exercise center fit into an overall theme that was buttressed by advertising designed to provide "a simple explanation of what values

Coors feels are important"—values that relate to its products, people, and work environment.

Perhaps the role of a corporate fitness center and how it combines with other socially responsible programs to contribute to corporate culture and identity was best summed up by Tenneco's J. L. Ketelsen. "It builds pride in our employees," he said. "They see us doing important, good things. It builds a culture of high morale. People are willing to come in and work hard, to create and do things because they recognize that the spirit is there in the company. . . . Building the fitness center is the single most gratifying thing I've ever done. The employees reacted to it with a spirit that was even better than we ever thought."

FITNESS PROGRAMS FOR EVERY COMPANY

While some corporations obviously have greater resources for employee programs than others, it doesn't take a multimillion-dollar facility or complicated plan to make an important difference. A basic employee health and fitness program can be set up by offering two or three benefits, including periodic physical examinations, communication about health risks, and low-cost exercise options.

1. Periodic Health Evaluations

Most larger companies offer their employees annual health evaluations. As a benefit, they're a given. The practice recognizes that, in the end, corporate health depends on individual health. I believe, however, that many companies are getting shortchanged on the results of periodic employee physical examinations. (I would also include preemployment evaluations in this category.)

All too often, the emphasis of these evaluations is to discover currently existing disease. This is an important function of a medical evaluation, of course, but the periodic evaluation by a physician can do much more. It can be an important time to intervene on negative habits, alert an employee to risk factors he or she might not have been aware of, and plan health-enhancing programs in weight loss, nutrition, and exercise.

If you as an individual or your company as an employer are not getting the kind of state-of-the-art thinking and performance that includes disease prevention, risk factor reduction, and life-style prescrip-

147

tion, in addition to disease detection, you should insist upon it, or find another health care provider. There is no question that the links between health, fitness, and performance so clearly evidenced by top executives can also be encouraged in middle managers and other employees, and the periodic health evaluation is an excellent place to start.

2. Risk Factor Reduction

Regardless of the size of your company, reduction in the risk of individuals in developing coronary heart disease (CHD) makes sense—in both human and economic terms. It is also the area where the best information and most reasonable, cost-effective programs are available.

Smoking Cessation

The multiple health problems associated with smoking are well documented—and clearly heeded by America's top executives. The incidence of cigarette smoking among those in our survey had plummeted to 10%, down from an estimated 25% to 30% as recently as 1980. Unfortunately, approximately 30% of the adult population in the United States and 29% of the work force still smoke cigarettes. Besides representing a major risk to the personal health of those who smoke, it also spells extra cost to your company in health care dollars. The additional direct, annual medical expenses that the average smoker costs a company are conservatively estimated to range between $300 and $800. The indirect costs may be considerably higher. Dow Chemical Company, for example, found that smokers average 5.5 more days of absence and 8 more days of disability leave each year than nonsmokers.

As the health hazards of exposure to smoke, or "passive smoking," become clearer, there will undoubtedly be even more pressure for employers to provide smoke-free environments. Laws in 10 states and 150 municipalities already restrict smoking in the workplace. Spurred by recommendations from the National Academy of Sciences, smoking has already been banned on flights lasting less than two hours and may soon be banned on all domestic airline flights.

The trend to restrict smoking in work environments is growing rapidly. The Bureau of National Affairs, a private research firm, reported that 36% of American corporations restricted smoking in 1986, with

23% more actively considering policies to limit smoking. This compares with 8% that limited smoking in 1981. In 1984, Boeing Company became the largest American company (85,000 employees) to ban smoking. Its statement to employees opened with the following words:

> After careful review and consideration of all the available information, the Boeing Company has decided to take some positive steps toward providing a smoke-free working environment for all employees. While no absolute date has been set for establishing a total prohibition on smoking, it is the intent of the company to do so.

When asked to comment on the policy, Boeing president Malcolm Stamler said, "It's the responsibility of management in any company to provide the cleanliest, safest, and most healthful environment for its employees. Boeing is continually striving to meet these objectives and developing a smoke-free environment is an essential ingredient.

"When we provide a better operating atmosphere for our high-tech machinery than we do for the people who operate it," Stamler continued, "then it's time to reassess policies—and that's what's been done."

The majority of *Fortune* 500 CEOs I talked with and virtually all of the *Inc.* 100 and *Venture* 100 CEOs had already restricted or banned smoking in the workplace or were contemplating doing so. The trend to create nonsmoking environments is particularly strong in entrepreneurial companies where the CEO is used to taking prompt action to change things he or she doesn't like.

One of the remarkable aspects of this trend is the description most CEOs give of how easy it was to implement a smoke-free environment. Most had anticipated considerable opposition. But, almost without exception, very little, if any, opposition materialized. The experience at Interand was not unusual. "We put an end to smoking in the workplace with the exception of one dungeonlike room in the extreme back of the building," explained CEO Leonard Reiffel. "And we offered all of our employees who are smokers reimbursement for going to smoking cessation clinics. I knew there would be resentment at the beginning, and there was some—one secretary and a consultant, both of whom smoked, left. But overall, the policy is going over very well. People have taken it as an opportunity to finally get over the top and stop."

Most surveys have shown surprisingly little opposition from smokers to well-planned schedules to restrict or ban smoking at work. Creating a smoke-free environment is one step that, for almost no expense, can make a major impact on the health and welfare of your employees and save money for the company at the same time. How should you take such a step? Start with a series of memos and announcements to all employees. Make a case for a smoke-free environment and give a clear timetable to accomplish it. The schedule may take six months to a year. As part of the program, offer employees optional—but reputable— smoking cessation programs both on- and off-site that are paid for, or at least partially supported by, the company. Such an approach couples implementation of a worthwhile policy with expression of concern for the health of all employees.

In short, creating a smoke-free environment is one of the best things you can do for your employees. To make the policy work, give ample notice ahead of time (at least 90 days), offer ways to help people stop, and apply it fairly at all levels of the company (executives, managers, and supervisors should not be allowed to smoke simply because they have private offices or cubicles).

Cholesterol Screening

As the data strongly linking elevated cholesterol levels to coronary disease continue to accumulate, there is increasing incentive to screen individuals for early detection of elevated cholesterol. This is an ideal type of program to offer executives and other employees. Your local hospital or clinical laboratory may be able to send a technician to your company. Portable cholesterol analyzers now allow cholesterol determinations to be performed on-site, in a matter of minutes. Your hospital or local chapter of the American Heart Association should be able to help you arrange the screenings. The cost is low and the potential benefits are immense.

Hypertension Screening

Multiple national education projects show that the work site is an excellent place to screen individuals for high blood pressure. If you have a corporate medical department, this should be easy to carry out. Alternatively, your local hospital will be happy to arrange for health professionals to come to your company for a morning, screen employees for high blood pressure, and distribute the excellent educational materials available from the American Heart Association.

There may also be a nearby major medical center or school that can provide a place for professionals to come and screen your employees for high blood pressure. To access the right people, call either the department of medicine or primary care at a nearby medical center.

It may be possible to combine cholesterol and blood pressure screening with one group of health care professionals. Many companies do this by conducting "health fairs" on one day every year.

3. Exercise Options

There are numerous alternatives for company exercise programs. They range from multimillion-dollar corporate fitness facilities such as those established by Coors, PepsiCo, and Tenneco, to partial copayment of membership fees in local clubs offered by many smaller entrepreneurial companies.

If your company has never offered an exercise program to its employees but would like to start, the best advice is to go slowly. Start with a simple, low-cost program, determine the level of participation, and then move to more sophisticated and elaborate programs if the level of interest is high—and your budget allows them.

One good way to start is by offering a couple of exercise classes taught by outside exercise specialists. These can typically be performed after-hours in existing space (many companies convert the cafeteria to an exercise area after work). Exercise specialists can be found at local recreational facilities.

Another good way to start a simple exercise program in your company is to build a couple of showers. This simple, relatively inexpensive amenity can make a big difference to your executives or other employees who want to go for a run or fitness walk during lunchtime. They will return refreshed and ready to give you more quality hours in the afternoon.

The next step—one taken by many small and medium-size companies—is to establish an exercise room on the premises. Typically the space for such a facility is small—200 to 400 square feet are sufficient. Modern exercise hardware such as multipurpose weight-training equipment, several stationary cycles, and a treadmill can easily fit into this amount of space. Expertise to equip such a room is available through most of the major exercise equipment manufacturers. Also, your local recreational facility can typically provide an exercise specialist to help you plan a small facility, as well as supervision several hours a day on a contract basis.

Facilities larger than a small exercise room generally require significant planning and capital expenditure. In 1981, for example, Nashua Corporation established an exercise facility in its plant. The in-house program includes aerobics and walking programs, exercise bikes, rowing machines, and even a swimming pool. If you are contemplating this level of commitment, advice can be obtained from the Association for Fitness in Business, a national corporate fitness and wellness organization based in Indianapolis, Indiana, and from the YMCA of the USA in Chicago or from one of its local branches. Many major medical centers have also developed the expertise to help you.

Beyond exercise options, other programs that can be offered to employees as part of corporate fitness or wellness include weight management, stress reduction, psychological and substance abuse counseling, and injury prevention and/or treatment (particularly avoidance of back injuries). All of these programs have merit, and which ones you choose should be governed by the unique needs and demands of your particular company. Before you make a commitment, just be sure to check the background of vendors offering these kinds of services. Many institutions, from hospitals to health clubs, are now heavily involved in these areas and can offer your company the kind of stable relationship and well-thought-out program that will be of most benefit to your employees.

PROGRAMS FOR SMALL BUSINESSES

Most examples of innovative corporate fitness programs come from the *Fortune* 500 giants. For obvious reasons, larger companies thus far have been the undisputed leaders in corporate fitness. Yet, small businesses offer an immense opportunity for creativity and innovation in health and fitness for their employees.

By sheer numbers, "small" enterprises dominate the American corporate scene. According to the Small Business Administration, there are 4.7 million small companies (between 2 and 500 employees) in the

United States. Constituting 99% of the total number of American businesses, these small firms employ more than half (58%) of the work force. More than 45% of the work force is employed by companies with between 2 and 100 employees. Moreover, during the 1980s, companies with fewer than 100 employees generated two-thirds of all new jobs in the United States. Though individually small in size, small businesses are big in terms of human resources and economic impact.

In our survey, 530 of the 1,139 respondents, or 47%, were chief executives of companies with less than 500 employees. As a group, these CEOs tend to be slightly younger than their counterparts among *Fortune* 500 and Dun's corporations (average age for small-company CEOs was 47; for large-company executives, 52). Most of their health and fitness practices, however, are similar to those of the overall sample: 90% pay attention to at least some aspect of their diet, 67% know their blood pressure, 65% exercise regularly, and only 11% smoke.

One theme that came up consistently in interviews with CEOs of small companies is the strong desire to implement a coherent corporate fitness strategy but great concern about its cost. Most had already implemented some of the basic strategies, such as establishing a smoke-free environment, but were struggling to determine which other programs would be appropriate for their company. With few exceptions, small businesses do not relate such programs to insurance coverage and health care cost control. Like their giant counterparts, they are much more likely to view fitness programs as vehicles for creating a positive work environment. When the U.S. Department of Health and Human Services surveyed the top fitness programs in small companies, the overwhelming majority reported that the major justification for their program was to improve human relations in the organization.

Two benefits of corporate fitness programs that have been consistently demonstrated are particularly relevant to small companies. First, such programs reduce absenteeism—a key issue in small companies, where "lean" staffing can mean that the absence of only one or two employees can dramatically decrease efficiency. Second, fitness programs clearly improve company morale—an aspect particularly prized in small companies where a "family atmosphere" is often highly valued and pursued.

Perhaps the greatest advantage that small companies have in instituting corporate fitness programs is the ability to respond quickly. Stockholders and bureaucracies aside, owners of small businesses can act swiftly, based on personal decisions, to implement policies that favor employee health and fitness. The specifics of such policies will vary considerably from company to company; however, as a starting point, there are several simple steps you can take. First, review your company employee policies (they should be in writing), practices, and physical environment. Simple provisions such as vending machines with fruits and juices (versus cigarettes or candy), a nonsmoking area for lunch or work breaks, and showers or a small exercise area can make a significant difference in employee morale and productivity. They also send a strong message about how the company feels about its employees.

Judith Kaplan, CEO of Action Products International, a $3.8-million souvenir wholesaler with 46 employees, started her own exercise program several years ago by working out regularly on an exercise gym. Recognizing its benefits, she set up a "nonsmoking" exercise facility at her company. "We have a whole room with a universal gym . . . twenty-two stations, bikes, mirrors, TV, videocassette," Kaplan reported, noting that the equipment manufacturer helped employees set up their own programs for use of the facility. "Anyone can use it, as long as they get an evaluation beforehand—they've got to know what levels they should start at, charts on how much weight to lift at first, and so forth."

In-house exercise equipment is not the only option, however, for small companies. There are other alternatives for those who find that space and/or budgets are just too tight. Some pay a portion of membership dues in local health clubs; others sponsor jogging or walking clubs. A few even retain a local exercise specialist two or three times a week to conduct exercise classes. Jacor Communications offers a cash bonus to employees who give up smoking for 60 days; those who quit smoking entirely earn $1,000 or a special vacation. Periodic screenings for cholesterol levels and high blood pressure can be offered, as well as smoking clinics and weight or stress-reduction classes. If your local hospital cannot help you institute such programs, contact a regional medical center or educational institution.

In short, company size needn't be a hindrance when it comes to providing a health and fitness program for employees. Small companies, in particular, depend on the individual effort, hard work, and creativity of their employees. The investment in commonsense programs that will improve their health and fitness will have direct and meaningful impact on their productivity.

COMMITMENT AT THE TOP

As I talked with top executives of companies of all sizes, from start-ups to *Fortune* 500 pacesetters, one thing became abundantly clear: The level of commitment of senior management, often the CEO, determines the company's level of commitment to corporate fitness. As Robert Rechholtz of Coors put it, "It always comes from the top. In any company, the climate is set by the CEO and his group of senior managers. In our company, the whole wellness priority was established by William Coors himself."

Tenneco's K. W. Reese offered a similar assessment of the role that J. L. Ketelsen played in creating his company's fitness program: "It keys off the leader. If J. L. Ketelsen was a nonexerciser, a smoker, or a hell-raiser, we wouldn't have the program we have today. He never tried to hide the fact that he had heart problems. Instead, he stepped up and said, 'I've had open heart surgery. I want a diet and exercise program, and I'm going to do everything I can to live as long as I can and enjoy it.' Then, using his position as chief executive, he began to make things happen—and to encourage all of us to get with it. First came the installation of a gym on the thirtieth floor—just a small room with a couple of treadmills and a few other pieces of equipment. Then came the idea of a fitness center. It was an opportunity for all of us and we knew it."

I have yet to encounter a case in which a significant corporate fitness program was instituted without the CEO's active support. Corporate fitness is not a monolith that requires a multimillion-dollar investment. In a matter of a few weeks, at relatively little cost, innovative practices and programs can be put in place that will have a long-term, positive impact on the health and fitness of your employees. The bottom line is that the buck stops with you. With your leadership, the links between health, fitness, and performance at the top can be translated from the executive office to a much wider sphere of individuals—the American work force.

8

View from the Top

What does it take to succeed as a CEO? There are several basic elements that should be in place. First, if you're married, you have to have the complete understanding of your wife that this is the life-style both of you want.

Second, you have to have a certain inner feeling that what you're doing is what makes you happy—or you'd better change it. If you don't like what you're doing, you've got more stress to start with than you can really handle.

Third, you have to recognize that the person who is working fifteen hours a day isn't necessarily the one who's doing the best job.

Other attributes? Don't try to take on every responsible action. It's a team effort. You have to work with people and delegate to those you trust. Finally, you have to have a disciplined rest period. Whether it's once a week or once a month—it will be different for different personalities and physical makeups—you need the discipline of just winding down.

—T. F. RUSSELL, chairman and CEO
Federal-Mogul Corporation

The detailed responses of the 1,139 top executives who answered our questionnaire provided a unique opportunity to take the physical pulse of the people who are running American business. Our follow-up interview provided a more in-depth picture of their corporate world view on topics ranging from the factors that contributed to their success and the attributes of a good manager to social and ethical responsibilities. It is this other aspect of corporate America—the visions and philosophies of its leaders—that form the basis of this chapter. Here we share their views of the performance side of the health and fitness equation.

REACHING PERFORMANCE GOALS

More than 97% of the executives who responded to our survey indicated at least one strategy or specific thing that they do to ensure they reach performance goals. Sixty-five percent checked off "work overtime"; 50%, "study and prepare"; and 46%, "work weekends." These were closely followed by exercise, eating properly, and following a planned program, all of which were listed by more than 40% of the executives. The least employed tactic, checked off by only 12% of the respondents, was "personal program for handling stress."

The average executive works a considerable 54 hours a week. While the executives we interviewed strongly emphasized that a person should be judged not by the number of hours worked but by the quality of his or her work, there nevertheless was equal emphasis on the fact that extraordinary results require extraordinary efforts. When asked to share his view of the most important contributing factor in his rise to the top position at Simon & Schuster, for example, Richard Snyder didn't hesitate a second: "Hard work. It's all got to do with that. Period. Nothing else. There are no shortcuts. There are a lot of guys pouring out of universities every year with similar IQs and backgrounds. The ones who are going to make it are the ones who are more diligent and dedicated and have high work standards."

Terry Jacobs, chairman of Jacor Communications, offered this advice to young executives starting out in entrepreneurial careers: "Perseverance is the most important thing. You have to be willing to work harder than you ever dreamed possible. You have to be willing to fight through times when it looks as if you just aren't going to make it. Don't give up and always keep an optimistic attitude. Stick at it long enough, and you'll find a way.

"I used to carry a quote from Longfellow in my pocket, which is now framed on my office wall. It's something I believe very strongly." Jacobs read the quote out loud:

> The heights by great men reached and kept
> Were not attained by sudden flight,
> But they, while their companions slept,
> Were toiling upward in the night.
>
> —HENRY WADSWORTH LONGFELLOW
> from *The Ladder of St. Augustine*

The ability to persevere long after others would have given up can be a double-edged sword for executives. On one side, it enables them to mount monumental efforts to accomplish a task. On the other, it can verge on the type of obsessive behavior that precludes other important activities, such as time out for family life, exercise, vacations, and even healthy meals.

Top executives are quick to emphasize the difference between working inordinately long hours and working effectively. As Winnebago's former president and CEO Gerald Gilbert put it: "The most successful executives are those who are energetic *and* can organize their lives best. They do their jobs in eight hours as opposed to twelve."

"There's a big difference between workaholics and people who work hard," noted Kenneth L. Otto, senior vice-president at Tenneco. "Workaholics are compulsive. The job becomes an obsession. They are constantly on the verge of crisis, constantly overwhelmed by what they're doing, and they end up not being very productive. Commitment to work is not unhealthy. You can work long hours without falling out of healthy habits that keep you productive."

In the end, the ability to set priorities and control work schedules is considered essential in meeting performance goals. "CEOs are used to controlling their workday. When I come in on Monday, I know what I'm going to do. I might get interrupted or sidetracked, but I'm pretty good at getting back to what I'm supposed to be doing and *should* be doing. I think that's extremely important," explained Medical Care International's Donald Steen.

"You just have to be careful that you don't let other people's schedules run your life," he continued. "For example, you can get into situations on the road where you catch an early morning plane, have lunch with a group, have a late dinner, check into a hotel, and catch an early flight the next morning. Unless you're a unique physical and mental specimen, it can really wear you down.

"A normal person has to be careful to say, 'I'm not going to meet at six-thirty A.M. if I've been up late the night before.' You can still work sixty hours a week but do it in such a way that you control when and how and don't end up a basket case."

The same discipline required to control work and travel schedules is applied to social functions. Numerous executives pointed out the importance of limiting the number of business-related invitations they accept. John Bierwirth, formerly of Grumman, offered this advice to young executives: "The extraneous, unnecessary demands on your time are what you have to watch out for. I think that people on the way up or near the top feel that they have to attend all the social functions. It's a great drain on their strength. The food and drink and cigarette smoke aren't good for their health—particularly when what they really get out of it is almost nothing. The ability to decide what to do with your time is as important an ability as there is in the game."

It's more than controlling time, it's also what executives do with their time. "Two things separate the men from the boys as you move up the corporate ladder," observed Joe B. Foster, former executive vice-president at Tenneco. "The first is the ability to set priorities—to see what's important and what's not. A lot of guys get tangled up in the details of a particular problem, but it just isn't that big a deal. They simply weren't able to see where their interest should have been directed.

"The second thing is the ability to handle more than one project at a time. At our level, you have to be able to deal with thirty or forty different problems. You might work on one for only two or three minutes and then you're off on another one. You have to find the most important problems to focus on, but still keep thirty or forty balls in the air."

Within the workday, most executives have developed strategies for controlling what they will and will not get involved in. A common problem is subordinates' demands on their time. As one CEO said, "The most important part of being a leader is not being pulled away from your vision by the day-to-day problems that should be handled by your staff. Everybody, on a daily basis, will want a chunk of your time and if you give it to them, you won't be able to perform your job—to set the overall direction for the company."

LUCK, TALENT, AND RISKS

Hard work and perseverance. Ability to set priorities and control time. What else contributes to executives' rise to the top? Are they born with an inherent drive to climb the ladder? Is it mainly intelligence? Street smarts? Experience? Luck? Taking risks when others won't?

A little bit of all of the above, in differing degrees, depending on the individual experience of the executive you are talking to. Said one: "I think it's something you are born with. I think it's in the genes. I've always had a desire to succeed from very early in life. There's a drive. I don't know. It's pride. It's desire. It's fear of failure. I'm cut out the way I am. Twenty-five years after I started in business, I still work through the lunch hour most of the time, not because I'm trying to prove anything. I just like to keep busy. I think it's the same thing that makes people successful in whatever they choose to do, whether it's entertainment or whatever."

Competitiveness, intelligence, and a desire to excel were frequently mentioned by top executives as qualities that contribute to success. Many, too, tipped their hat to lady luck. "One key to success is having some ability—the ability to think. I don't think there's any substitute for that," stated Foster. "But beyond that, being in the right place at the right time is critical in anybody's career in a corporation and anyone who tells you that they did it on sheer ability is bullshitting you.

"At least at one point in your career, you have to be where the major interest of the corporation is at that time. Once that happens, you can achieve recognition for your contributions and have some control over what's going on in the company. I was fortunate to be sent to Louisiana when we first began our offshore operations back in the late fifties. I attracted some attention and have had good assignments ever since. There's an element of luck in anything that happens in life and that certainly applies to corporate careers."

Foster referred to the saying, "You can't win if you're not at the table." And added: "Lucky people are the ones who are at the table. And if you're there, you've got a good chance of lightning striking."

"Absolutely there's an element of luck," agreed Navistar's board member and former CEO Donald Lennox. "Look at the odds of becoming a CEO of one of the *Fortune* 1,000 companies, for example. There must be a hundred thousand executives in this country today who are qualified to have those thousand jobs. It's just that they got in behind the wrong person—just the luck of the draw.

"When I retired from Xerox at the end of 1980, I had had a successful business career," Lennox continued, explaining his own encounter with luck. "I had always performed well in the various assignments I had and rose progressively. But I just wasn't in the right spot at the right age to be considered for the top. So if I hadn't made the move to International Harvester to help out for a while, I would have wound up just having retired from Xerox and sort of drifting off into oblivion. It just so happened I came in here and when the men in the two top positions left in 1982, the board asked me to take the top position on. Luck!"

For executives in smaller companies or entrepreneurial companies, being at the table is not so much being in the right job at the right time as it is knowing when to make a bet. "My definition of luck is when preparation meets opportunity—being able to recognize opportunities and being willing to take risks to go after them," said Jacobs. "That's how I have been successful. If you put in long hours and take the risks involved, it's amazing how lucky you can get."

The ability to take risks, whether for an entrepreneur like Jacobs or in career paths in larger corporations, is viewed as an essential characteristic of the successful executive. Charles Clough, president, CEO, and chairman of Nashua Corporation, summed it up very succinctly: "You have to be willing to take risks if you are going to get out ahead of the pack."

In fact, taking chances is fundamental to the business-learning process. "You have to have enough inner strength to go out and try to win in business. There are a lot of people in this world who, quite honestly, just don't have the willingness to take the chance of losing. But if you are willing to go out and stick your neck out and try to win a project, make a sale, or whatever, you will gradually learn how to do it better, how to present your position better, and you will end up succeeding," advised John Bierwirth.

"People who play it safe take the greatest risks," noted Kenneth L. Otto. "Intelligent risk takers develop security. If we spent half as much time learning how to take risks as we do trying to avoid them, we wouldn't fear so much. Security, like happiness, often eludes those who pursue it most."

In a similar vein, Interand's Leonard Reiffel observed: "I get enormous satisfaction out of doing something hard and committing myself to it, and hopefully doing it well. I have great sadness for people who go through life unwilling or afraid to commit themselves. They're afraid that if they throw themselves into a somewhat corrosive atmosphere, they might dissolve. There is only a very short time on this earth, and you may as well become part of the passions of the times."

Apart from luck, talent, and risks, many executives shared specific strategies or approaches that they believe contribute to success. One of the most frequently mentioned is what might be called the First Corporate Commandment: Know Thy Job. "Whatever job you're in, you have to figure out what the important leverage of that job is. Usually it's not exactly what the job title implies or the routine things you do every day. You get a job description, but even that doesn't really tell you what it is about your job that contributes to the welfare and progress of the company. Figure that out. Then do it very well," recommended Dean Freed, vice-chairman of EG&G.

Looking back at his career at Fruehauf, Robert Rowan described what might be called the Second Corporate Commandment: Honor Thy Boss. "One of my goals was to make the man I worked for look as good as I possibly could. I must admit that I worked for three or four individuals who I thought were the biggest jerks I'd ever met. But I made a rule for myself. If I could help my boss, I was helping myself. Sometimes it took a while, but in the long run it proved successful. I would certainly give that advice to any junior executive starting today— the way to succeed is by making sure that the boss succeeds."

Implicit in the Honor Thy Boss rule is always be ready to take his place. "Some people get lucky and they're not ready. They miss an opportunity and luck goes right on by. I always tried, at least mentally, to do my boss's job. You have to think about how you would do it if you were he. Do your homework and be ready if the opportunity arises," said Tenneco's chairman and CEO J. L. Ketelsen.

But don't be in too much of a hurry. Several CEOs noted that a common mistake made by junior executives is that they expect advancement too soon and often end up job-hopping and losing the momentum they had gained at their old firms. As Donald Lennox observed: "Too many young managers look to an established career path and plan their moves by a set time frame. So if they haven't gotten to a certain level in a company by a certain time, they start looking elsewhere. It's unfortunate because it often hurts their careers in the long run."

Dean Freed was more blunt in his advice to junior executives: "The first thing I'd say is forget everything you've ever heard and timetables and how many years it should take to be a vice-president, and so forth. Don't worry about it."

Counseled Ketelsen: "If you work hard and use your talents to the utmost of your abilities, something will happen. Be a team player; don't worry too much about your own career. Assume that if you do well and work toward the benefit of the company, good things will happen. Good work does not go unnoticed. You don't have to be out using your own muscle, tooting your own horn."

162

MANAGING

All of the contributing characteristics and advancement strategies in the world would not have gotten the top executives to where they are without exceptional management skills. Here the first and most important theme that emerged in our interviews was: Know Thyself.

"You have to be willing to take a clear look at yourself and understand your impact on other people," said Norton's vice-president of human resources Thomas Hourihan. "It's all well and good to talk about brilliant researchers or entrepreneurs, but the basic job of a manager is to manage people. And in order to manage people, you first have to learn how to manage yourself. You have to understand your strengths and weaknesses and work on areas where you need more strengths."

Part of this self-knowledge is the recognition that it takes more than just an individualistic drive to succeed to get to the top. "I've always been motivated by a drive to reach what I think are my own potentials and a drive to be number one. I carry that through virtually anything I do. However, it's essential to couple this kind of drive with feelings for other people. I don't think that anyone could get to the top of any organization unless he has a genuine sympathy for other people," observed Gerald Gilbert, former president and CEO of Winnebago Industries.

Over and over again, executives emphasized that the real key to success, and the one that causes some of even the most capable executives to flounder, is interpersonal skills. "I've been in situations where I've hired very brilliant people and then ended up firing them because they couldn't work well with others. It's extremely important to learn to get along with people and to understand what motivates them," said Jacobs.

"I don't think I'm necessarily smarter than anybody else or my talents are better than anybody else's. But I do think that the ability to motivate people and to get them to work together has contributed to my success more than anything else."

An essential part of interpersonal skills is learning to consult others in the management process. The old image of the unapproachable, autocratic CEO alone in his office single-handedly making decisions and charting the course of the company is rarely true any longer. "The biggest mistake anybody in this type of job can make is to try to do it all alone. It can't be done. You have to reach out and be willing to admit that you don't have all the answers," said Nashua Corporation's Charles Clough.

"The most successful people I've seen are good decision-makers. They take the time—whether it is a personnel decision or buying or selling a company—to carefully solicit the views of not just subordinates but also people who have knowledge and expertise they don't have. Some people's opinions may be more important to them than others, but they know they have to be objective about that, too. In the words of Kipling, 'Let all men count, but none too much.'" said Norton's Thomas Hourihan.

"Some executives are cosmetic in seeking others' views," he continued. "You know they've already made their minds up. The good decision-makers are not just consensus takers. They are sincere in soliciting opinions and discussing contrary opinions."

It's more than just making decisions. Teamwork is essential in the day-to-day management of a company—and the more so the larger the company. "In a company as big as Tenneco, in most of the *Fortune* 500 companies, it's difficult for a lone wolf to operate. You don't get things done as a lone wolf. You get things done through other people. Senior management's job is to set the priorities and work with other people as a team to get those projects done," noted Joe B. Foster.

Xerox president Paul Allaire agreed: "In a large corporation, I don't think a lone wolf would ever get promoted. You have to have the support of your colleagues. You have to show that you can manage an organization. You have to show that you are a team player. There's absolutely no question about it."

Successful teamwork depends on subordinates' respect for senior management and, in turn, senior management's concern for developing subordinates' potential. Tenneco's K. W. Reese summed up the sentiment of many top executives: "It's very important that you've gotten to the top in a professional way, that you've done it with class, that you haven't stepped over people or hurt them. And when you get to the top or close to the top, then you try to work with people and train them and give them the benefit of your experience—try to bring them along and develop them.

"If I were to retire tomorrow and someone were to ask me what I am most proud of, I could say a lot of different things—selling a business for one-and-a-half billion dollars, doing this deal or that deal, putting money in the bank for Tenneco. But the thing I'm most proud of is the many people I've trained who now hold key jobs in the company."

Norton's Hourihan characterized his approach to developing the careers of staff members this way: "When I delegate, I take vicarious pleasure watching people develop and do the things I used to do. In a way, it's like managing a baseball team. You don't hit the ball anymore, you name the lineup. They've got to have fun. They get the credit when they help the team. You're the manager and the buck stops at your door, but you have to encourage them to grow and be proud of their achievements.

"There's a certain amount of unselfishness that has to go along with it. You have to watch your ego. You can't sort of backhandedly say, 'He's done a great job,' and then whisper, 'but I really helped him do it all along.' You have to take genuine pleasure in the success of the people who work with you. Once they understand that and see you as a resource, they begin to say, 'He's an OK kind of guy.' "

At the same time, as Hourihan and other executives pointed out, there's a fine line between the ability to be liked by subordinates and commanding their respect. "There are times when you have to spell it out, what you're unhappy about, and it requires a little distance. What it comes down to is you'd like to get the affection along with the respect, but you'll take the respect first. Even when you do have to distance yourself, you feel that at least you've been honest. You've been objective. You've tried to help them look at themselves and improve themselves."

There is also the problem of the subordinate who is reluctant to level with the boss. "One of the worst people I can have working for me is a yes person. He's dangerous because he does just that—tells you what he thinks you want to hear, and you end up making decisions on fallacious data. What a successful manager needs is someone who will look him in the eye and say, 'I'll do it if you want me to do it that way, but I think it's a dumb goddamn idea.' You have to create an environment where your people know that you want them to tell you what they think," explained Navistar's Lennox.

"We'll discuss the idea and I might say, 'You're right. You saved me from making a mistake and let's modify it.' Or, after I've heard him out, I still may not think it's a dumb idea. When he leaves my office, I expect him to be satisfied that the problem has been straightened out, and I expect him to do exactly what we agreed to do."

A key ingredient is that certain leadership quality that elicits loyalty. "When you're dealing with a big company or organization, what you're trying to do is get a whole group of people to follow the vision of where you want to take them. Charisma is part of it, but it goes beyond that," observed John Nelson, chairman and CEO of Norton Company. "We had a CEO here who could call me into his office and say, 'I'm going to cut your pay ten percent,' and make me feel good about it. A certain kind of warmth and charm just came through. Is that valuable? I think it's critical."

Executives in smaller, entrepreneurial firms face different types of managerial challenges than their counterparts in larger corporations. Typically, the senior management staff—if there is one—is smaller, and each executive is called upon to take responsibility for various functions as the company grows. A common dilemma for a founder/CEO is the realization that the company has grown too big to manage alone or with just a few people. Some establish a management team by internal promotions; others hire from outside. It is not uncommon for the entrepreneur himself to step aside. Avner Parnes described his own replacement at MBI Business Centers: "I brought in a guy from IBM who'd been there twenty-five years, a real experienced guy used to managing three or five thousand employees, not six hundred like I had. He's a great communicator, a good manager, and he understands priorities better than I. I told everybody, 'He's much better than I am, guys, that's the reason I brought him in.' You have to understand those things. Nothing wrong with that. I believe, at least, that I can recognize my strengths and my weaknesses."

While Parnes described stepping aside as a "total relief," other entrepreneurs find relinquishing sole decision-making power and authority difficult. Said one: "It was very hard to let go, but we had reached a size where it became a matter of survival—both for me and the company. I finally realized that I had to structure the business and get it under control or it would eat me alive."

Some entrepreneurs simply have no interest in managing after their companies reach a certain size. As Carol Cone, president of a burgeoning five-year-old Boston public relations firm, observed: "Any entrepreneur worth his or her salt realizes that there will be a day when the reins must be handed over to someone who understands the mid-life of a company's existence. Mitch Kapor stepped down to Jim Manzi because he believed Lotus just wasn't the same anymore. Companies get to the size where they need different levels of management skills, and it is no longer fun for the entrepreneur. Entrepreneurs like to build things; they don't like to be the caretakers in the mid-life of a company's growth and have to pay attention to all the details. They want to be creating, not maintaining.

"An entrepreneur is someone who doesn't want to work for someone else. Someone who wants to set his or her own path. Entrepreneurs move to a different drummer."

MENTORS AND ADVISORS

An often-overlooked ingredient in an executive's rise to the top is the role of senior advisors and mentors. All of the executives we interviewed had at least one mentor, and many had three or four, who helped shape their careers and business philosophies. Observed Winnebago's Gilbert: "I had been moving along at a fairly decent pace when I went to work for a guy who was a vice-president at Control Data. As he moved forward in his career, he moved me right along with him. He certainly became my mentor and greatly speeded up my progression." Gilbert added: "Contacts are important. A lot of people have gotten their jobs more through their contacts than their capabilities."

"The greatest experience I had was working for Carl Linder," said Terry Jacobs. "If not the greatest entrepreneur, he was certainly one of the greatest ever in this country. He dropped out of school in the eighth grade and started with a little general store in a suburb of Cincinnati and built a corporation, American Financial Corporation, that's got assets of about nine billion dollars now.

"He taught me how to do my homework and how to outwork most other people. He's a hard worker. And he treats people well. He's rewarded people who helped him along the way. His employees have always shared in the wealth, and I have adopted that philosophy at Jacor. We have incentives, stock ownership plans, stock purchase options for our employees. I feel strongly that having employees share in the company's success makes you even more successful than if you tried to keep it all to yourself."

Sometimes mentors end up becoming trusted outside advisors. "I had more than one mentor, there were at least four or five people who helped shape my career and were instrumental in the success I've had," reported Fruehauf's Robert Rowan. One was Max Fischer, who was on our board for many years and whom I still regard highly. Occasionally when I have a problem that I need help with I'll call Max and say, 'Max, can you have lunch?' He has always been a tremendous help."

While all of the executives strongly advocate including senior management in day-to-day decision making, they also, like Rowan, have certain people they seek out for advice. Explained Donald Lennox: "I have found that it is helpful to have as sounding boards distinguished individuals who, because of their position or age or whatever, do not consider themselves as your possible successor or perhaps don't see themselves advancing very far beyond where they already are. Yet, because of their good common sense, you can use them to discuss contemplated moves or personnel shifts and they lend a different perspective on your ideas."

Outside business associates who share common problems and outlooks are also trusted advisors, particularly for CEOs in smaller or entrepreneurial companies. "I have evolved some very strong friendships and business relationships along the way where my success has been able to contribute to their success and theirs to mine," noted Jacobs. "It's important to develop relationships with people of a like mind who share your dream. Two heads are very often much better than one and three are better than two. I really believe that."

WOMEN EXECUTIVES

Although an overwhelming percentage of the respondents to our survey were men, interviews with several female CEOs provided insights into some of the issues women executives face. All agreed that while many of the pressures involved in managing a business are the same regardless of gender, some subtle—and not so subtle—differences exist.

One common issue is launching a successful career and raising a family. "A unique health hazard for women in business is making enough time to be with a family. Many women are putting off getting married and having families and, in fact, I advise young women not to get married until they are thirty so that they can better understand themselves and build their careers first," said Carol Cone. "Any woman who is going to advance has to work sixty to eighty hours a week. It is difficult, if not impossible, to be married and have children and work that many hours. Yet a woman is not going to advance unless she puts in that amount of time."

Several male CEOs looked back at their own early careers and wondered how a woman could possibly put in the amount of effort required to move ahead and still maintain a semblance of family life. One CEO in a company with an outstanding reputation for hiring and promoting women said candidly: "I look at the feminist movement and I find it in some aspects good but in other aspects just ridiculous. They expect a woman to be a CEO, a mother, and a lover, and all the things that go with that. You just can't do it successfully."

Once a woman has started a family, balancing business and parental responsibilities is a significant challenge. Lin Patterson, president and CEO of Appleton & Lange, described a situation earlier in her career that sums up how she views this dual responsibility. "My daughter got meningitis when my first business plan was due for Appleton. I went and stayed with her in the hospital. I brought along the business plan and it ended up that I could do that, too. But there was no question about what was going to come first. I've always put my children first. Most businessmen have wives to take care of situations like that. Maybe a man who was a single parent would have done the same thing I did."

Emergencies such as the one Patterson faced are one thing. Judith Kaplan, CEO of Action Products International pointed to the day-to-day pressures of running an entrepreneurial business and maintaining family responsibilities. "You have the classic working mother's syndrome. You're frequently at the office when you should be at home, and when you are at home, you're thinking of the office. Finally, I told myself that wherever I am at a certain time, I had to try to 'be' there. I guess that's what Eastern religions mean when they talk about living in 'this second.' But the truth is that it's easier said than done."

Do women CEOs react to stressful situations differently than men do? Here we got a variety of opinions. Lin Patterson expressed the prevailing view: "By the time a woman gets to the level of president or CEO of a company, she doesn't generally react any differently than a man would. I've seen men react extraordinarily emotionally to situations—very defensively. And I've seen women react that way, too."

However, Patterson noted that there may be some differences in the way women relate to subordinates: "Women executives may get more attached to people and, if so, I consider that a plus. I am very loyal to the

169

people I've brought into this company. If there's anything that motivates me to work hard, it's that I want to create a good working environment for them and help them succeed. Of course, you work hard to make a profit, too. Otherwise you wouldn't stay on the job. But the other part, the caring part, is more important to me."

For Carol Cone of Cone Communications, the caring part has its pluses, but it can also have its minuses. "Women are more emotional. It's in their makeup. They are more caring. They care about their employees and what their employees think of them. They are more humane. When they make decisions, they think about how they will affect people's lives overall," she noted. "But the emotion has to be kept in check. Sometimes instead of stepping back and being cool and really analyzing a situation, women respond on a more emotional basis. You have to be aware of your emotions and look at a problem rationally in terms of what's best for your organization."

Cone believes the women executives in her organization often "outshine the men in many situations" for a number of reasons. "Women are much better, across the board, in paying attention to detail. They are highly dependable when it counts. Women also have much less ego involvement in their interactions with peers. They're less back-stabbing at the senior levels. They are much more willing to negotiate and be flexible. I think women work better with men because there is less ego confrontation."

As all of the executives we interviewed noted, the increasing number of women in senior management positions has led to a breakdown in many of the old sexist stereotypes and communication barriers in the workplace. Still, some things may be slow to change. "I relate very well to the men in our company and they relate well to me. Sometimes, though, I think it's easier to relate to other women. Just like men find it easier to relate to other men. That's one of the reasons I think women are held back—it's easier to talk to a person of the same sex. It isn't an issue of sexuality; it's cultural, traditional," observed Patterson.

The women executives we interviewed never considered allowing themselves to be "held back" in their careers, even if it meant changing jobs in the face of discrimination; they simply lived up to what they felt was their potential in the business world. What they share most with their male counterparts is determined commitment to hard work and a drive to succeed. And all felt they had it in them from childhood. "My athletic background contributed tremendously to my business success," said Cone. "I rode horses and showed competitively from age seven. I played field hockey in junior high school and high school. I've skied from an early age. I carried the preparation and excitement and self-confidence into my business career.

"Athletics teach you how to be in touch and how to win and lose. I'm a fierce competitor; I love to win. And what is fun is the whole process of making the win happen. Sometimes when we are pitching a new business, people in the company will start talking about, 'If we win.' I correct them and say, 'No, not *if, when* we win.' In my mind, we've already won the business, and we just have to go through the process."

For Patterson, athletics also played an important role. "Sports have always been important to me. . . . I was a tomboy. I played baseball and football and everything else with the boys. I was very good at sports. It gave me a lot of confidence in myself. I never thought of myself as inferior or not being able to do something I wanted to do."

Like Cone and Patterson, Action Products's Kaplan realized early on that she had the drive to cut her own career path. "You have to want to have control over what you are doing, what you want the world to do. You don't want to get bored. When I was young, I'd get bored doing the same functional jobs. When I was just out of high school and going to college at night, I went for an interview for a job testing blood samples in a laboratory. Sure, I'd like to think I could have become a scientist. But all the job involved was three simple steps I had to do over and over again.

"The most important thing about being an entrepreneur is that you can't afford to get bored. You have to keep changing and enjoy every change. You have to want to do something better. You need the vision that you are going to accomplish something, even if it's just to prove to yourself that you can do it."

Kaplan described frustrating job experiences she had in the early 1960s. "I was looking for better jobs. I wanted to earn good money. I'd look at the ads in the *New York Times* and if I was qualified, I'd call up to make an appointment for an interview. I'd be told, 'Well, that job's for a man.' I kind of accepted that back then.

"I had a job where I went to my boss and said that as inventory control and traffic manager, I should be making as much as the guy who was packing and shipping—it was a very simple job, and he was making more than I was. My boss said, 'He's a man.' I said, 'What does that have to do with it?' He said, 'Well, some day he's going to have to support a

171

family.' The guy wasn't even married. I was very frustrated because it was clear I should have been earning more."

Kaplan then went through what she calls "turning on the light bulb." She read about and identified with many of the points the feminist movement was making about women on the job and realized, "It's not me and my capabilities. It's the world out there. I felt as if I were involved in a major movement. I kept trying to do more and do it better. It helped me along, some of the role models. Women who put their noses to the grindstone on whatever they felt strongly about, and just kept at it. Susan B. Anthony worked all her life, and she said that 'failure is impossible.' I believe that. You keep at it again and again and you can't get discouraged."

What of the future for women in business? "Today's businesswomen are untraditional," observed Cone. "They need men who are supportive and who are willing to share family responsibility. All the old rules are being broken. The former roles for women—what is acceptable in raising children, for example—must change if women are going to be leaders.

"Women have to accept the changes and so do men. We are only at the beginning of that. I believe that in twenty or thirty years, when there is a business environment that has fifty percent women at the top versus seventy-five percent of women at the bottom, the entire climate of the business world will change—and for the better."

What advice would these women executives offer to those starting out in the business world? "One of the key things is to pick a good boss to start with, someone who appreciates what you do and treats you appropriately. If you are in a situation where you feel there is a lot of resistance, leave and find another place," counseled Patterson. "I feel very strongly that you have to maintain your self-respect, your own integrity, whatever that means for you."

Cone had this advice for budding entrepreneurs: "For women or men, it's the same advice. You have to be driven. You have to be energetic. You have to have a niche, a product, or a service, that is unique and the confidence that you can sell it and move toward fulfilling a vision. You have to be incredibly stubborn and persistent. I compare it to being like one of those 'Bozo' punching bags that a lot of us had as children. You keep trying to knock it over, but there's a weight or sand in the bottom and it keeps bouncing back again and again. That's what it's like being an entrepreneur. If you can't bounce back up again and again, then you shouldn't do it because you'll get run over a lot."

BROADER SOCIAL CONCERNS

The emphasis executives place on the value of human relationships in motivating subordinates extends into larger social and human concerns through outside projects their companies get involved in. "When you get to be a chief executive officer, you can make things happen. You can move a whole organization and maybe a whole community," said Tenneco's Ketelsen. "I can get my kicks by having a bigger market share in tractors, which is a specific business item, or I can get my kicks by having sixteen hundred Tenneco employees involved in volunteer activities in community projects in and around Houston, as we do. I'm proud of that. It gives you great personal satisfaction to know that you're running an enterprise with that many people wanting to help others."

On a broader scale, Ketelsen observed: "I think most major corporations whose names are respected are involved in society. There are damn few that are not participating. . . . Some of the best minds in this country go into business. The leaders of American business are quite unique and capable. Having some of those minds work on social problems is very important. They don't have all the answers, but there's got to be interaction between business and government and organizations working on solving social problems. It's in the best interest for the future of business and our country."

For many executives, there's a personal dimension to their community involvement. Terry Jacobs described his work with children in community athletic programs and how it relates to his own childhood; he grew up pretty much on his own after his father died when he was nine years old. "Along the way there were people willing to help me. There was a football coach or friend's father or somebody who was involved in an organization I was part of. They took a little bit of extra time and spent extra effort to make me feel like I was a decent human being. It was important and made a lasting impression when someone showed extra kindness. I have always remembered that and have tried to do the same for others."

In many ways, the high level of social responsibility felt by top business leaders mirrors their high sense of personal and professional integrity. When asked about the issue of ethics and the popular image of finagling businessmen who are interested only in wealth and power, all of the executives we interviewed literally bristled with indignation. "Business leaders even in the most competitive industries operate with the highest level of integrity," said one CEO. "That's why it's so repulsive that executives are characterized that way. You know you're going to be in a certain business for the rest of your life, so you're not going to try to screw other people."

"The people I do business with are ethical people. They really don't differ in the way they approach life and their personalities from other kinds of people. They have high ethics, family concerns, and integrity," echoed another CEO.

These top executives feel very strongly that the main source of their image problem is that they have been indiscriminately lumped in the public eye with the "insider" Wall Street scandals. "We all get blurred. We all get painted with the same brush," noted Ketelsen. "You know, you can't even paint Wall Street with the same brush because there are some very, very high-quality people operating there who aren't involved in that sort of thing. They're doing an honest job, but they get painted, too. The people running industrial corporations or corporate entities involved in the productive process have a high level of ideals and standards."

This is not to suggest that executives are free of ethical dilemmas, particularly when the decisions they make in the interest of corporate profits affect the livelihoods of many people. It is to say, however, that they don't take such actions lightly and spend considerable time analyzing the moral and ethical implications. It's hardest, as Donald Lennox pointed out, when you get into "gray" areas.

"In my experience," he noted, "I have not found any lack of corporate ethics in the basic black-and-white areas of ethical behavior. Where I believe we need to do a lot more work is in the gray areas. Take us, for example. We're a good, profitable company, and we decide that rather than spend a lot of money to rehabilitate an old plant in Ohio, we'll pay a little more money and go down to South Carolina in a union-free, right-to-work area where labor is cheaper and eventually we'll save a lot of money. In that Ohio town, we have meant a lot to the people and have been a big part of the tax base. I believe we have an ethical and moral responsibility to take certain actions with respect to those people and that town."

Top executives are just as adamant about the charge that they are out for personal financial gain as they are about the question of ethics. "Money is a satisfier, not a motivator," summed up the executive vice-president of a *Fortune* 500 company. "You've got to pay a guy competitive wages so he knows he's doing as well as his peers. But that's not what drives me. What drives me is getting things done."

WHAT ABOUT FATHER TIME?

One final concern among the top executives was the realization, at a certain age and a certain point in their careers, that it was time to plan ahead for their own future. "I'm realistic. I'm in my mid-fifties. People in my position always think down the road because that's the key to the job—planning," said one executive. "When I became CEO ten years ago, I didn't have a long-range plan. But eventually you start to say you want to combine what you're doing with a satisfying personal life. That's one of the benefits of age—you've experienced a lot of things and you understand the value of thinking ahead."

Whether or not they have made definite plans for when they will retire or what they will do after retirement, all of the executives know one thing for sure—they do not want to become inactive. "I would like to think that I could work well into my sixties and maybe into my seventies, but in the corporation that just doesn't happen. You have to make room for somebody else to come along. But I can't picture the day when I'm down on the Cape just going to get the paper and having coffee and doughnuts and killing time before I tee off. Just talking about that scares me. I mean, I'd love to do that for two weeks, but not forever," said Norton's Hourihan. "So I'm looking at the next phase of my life, which says I'm going to have to do something with myself after Norton Company. Something intellectually stimulating. I know I'll have to keep myself in good shape because I've seen too many people become too sedentary in their late fifties and early sixties. I have this image of six years from now, or whenever I leave this company, of being into something new where I can use my experience and wisdom and be vigorous enough to carry on a very active workweek, and where I can call the tune on the rest of my life."

Time and again, we heard the words, ". . . but I will never really retire." Said one executive: "To me, sitting still would be a form of dying. I'll stay here another six or seven years or as long as I feel I can do the job and not be blocking someone else's progress. But I've already started thinking about some companies I want to start up in my sixties and seventies."

Other executives said they intend to teach and do consulting work after they leave their companies. A few want to try their hand at writing. And most, like Hourihan, emphasized that they intend to keep up their regular exercise programs to maintain their energy and vigor for the next stage in their lives.

Tenneco's K. W. Reese described his future agenda: "I'm fifty-seven now; if I go on to sixty-five depends on whether or not I'm still able to contribute. At the point I can't contribute and feel I'm blocking other people from running the company the way it ought to be run, I'll move on. But I'll never really retire. I'm very active in many other things, with the University of Houston, the Better Business Bureau, the hospital. . . . I'm on three boards and would like to maybe increase that by a couple. Those types of things are very time-consuming and will keep me moving and interested. I don't ever intend to stop enjoying life. I'd like to do more traveling with my wife.

"But the main thing is, if you come back and see me when I'm sixty-five—if I'm retired at that time—I think what you'll find is that I'm getting out of bed at five-thirty or six o'clock, running four, five, or six miles, depending on how I feel. And the rest of the day I'm doing something leisurely like swimming, playing tennis, golfing, boating, or whatever, and trying to keep my wife from spoiling the grandkids too much."

For many chief executives, the final stages of their careers involve a sense of personal and professional fulfillment in a job well done, in making an impact that will last. Observed one CEO: "Once you get to the top level, all of the responsibility is yours, and your aspirations change slightly. You want to leave a legacy. It's not the next promotion that matters, but leaving a legacy so that the historians, whoever they may be, will say, 'During his tenure, good things happened.' "

For the here and now, Richard Snyder summed up the feeling of many executives: "I don't dwell on it, but I'm certainly aware that I'm past the halfway mark. Only a fool wouldn't appreciate that. So you begin to think—how many good years are left? I make a point of enjoying my job. I don't think you'll ever meet a CEO who doesn't enjoy what he does."

Epilogue

What's the point of doing something if it overshadows everything else in your life? You have to mix the realization that it takes tremendous effort to succeed with some good judgment, otherwise you end up seeing only trees and no forest. You can't just say you'll work five days a week, because there will be a guy down the street who's working seven days a week, and he'll eat your lunch.

You have to ask yourself, "Am I willing to do that job in the first place? And if I am, what balance can I put in there so I don't become obsessed with it?" Personally, I think a good exercise program is the best way to balance it out.

—RONALD THOMAS, chairman and former president
    Ciprico, Inc.

I am sitting in my study in Newton, Massachusetts, about to lift weights and work out on my stationary cycle. This morning I ran Heartbreak Hill along the Boston Marathon route for what is probably the four hundredth time in the past two years. Earlier this afternoon, I finished the final chapter of this book—the culmination of more than two years of intense work. During that time, I wrote consistently, often 3,000 to 4,000 words a day. I also increased my workout schedule from once to twice a day, a luxury usually restricted to weekends.

Why do I increase my workout routine when I'm under pressure and have less free time to exercise? When we correlated the results of our survey in terms of hours worked, stress levels, and exercise patterns, the findings rang true to my experience. Those who work longer hours are those who exercise more regularly. This conclusion mirrored the results of a previous survey of more than 300 top executives and salesmen at a major computer company. In that survey, those who worked more than 60 hours a week were *twice* as likely to have regular exercise programs as those who worked less than 50 hours a week. Further, those who exercised regularly were significantly less likely to view their jobs as stressful

177

compared to the nonexercisers or intermittent exercisers. The question is not one of time; it's one of priorities.

There is no question that fitness and performance are inexorably linked to each other in my own life. I claim no originality in this notion. Intuitively or cognitively, it has fueled the daily habits of thousands of adults who jog, fitness walk, or aerobic dance on a daily basis. Human beings simply feel better, look better, and perform better when they are active.

Under the best of circumstances, adhering to a lifelong exercise program is not easy. Even avid exercisers often experience difficulty sticking to their regimens. The challenge is particularly difficult for managers whose lives are typically marked by constant time pressures and interruptions. Numerous executives I've seen in my practice and many of those interviewed for this book have experienced periods in their lives when they felt they were simply "too busy" for a fitness program. Most discovered in short order, however, that exercise was essential in maintaining their performance and active life-styles.

The best advice? Accept the reality of the challenge—it *is* difficult to stick with a lifelong exercise program—and meet it head-on, much as you do in dealing with daily business problems. Develop strategies to keep you going. Schedule exercise sessions into your day like any other important business appointment. Choose exercises you like. Work out with colleagues or friends. Keep a log, and reward yourself periodically.

If you are just starting an exercise program, focus on the first six months. Statistically, once you make it through that period your chances of carrying on the program for a lifetime improve dramatically. In the end, it comes down to self-discipline and, even more important, planning. As one CEO noted, "If you don't plan for exercise, it won't happen."

More than any other segment of society, America's top executives are acutely aware of the link between their health and fitness practices and their performance. It was to explore the nature of these links that we began this journey. As the project progressed, it became clear that the image of the impersonal, hard-nosed executive is very different from what I was seeing and hearing. Here were people running some of the country's largest corporations, wrestling daily with complex decisions that frequently affect thousands of lives. Yet their lives were not complicated at all. In fact, they made great efforts to keep life simple. Love, trust, and concern for their families, subordinates, employees, and communities were much in evidence. As I discovered in the executives' often touching and inspiring responses to my questions, people don't reach the "top" by stepping over bodies.

I have derived great personal and professional satisfaction from watching medical and scientific knowledge on health and fitness grow over the past few years. And we've only begun to scratch the surface. In the future, we will see more specific, concrete links between exercise and cardiovascular health, improved cholesterol levels, resistance to colds, increased longevity, and perhaps even a reduction in cancer. We will also see a better understanding of the interface between mind and body. Experience tells us that we feel better and think more clearly when we exercise. Future research will begin to tell us why and how this happens. In the meantime, I hope the dialogue with executives will continue and together we can explore those uncharted linkages between health, fitness, and daily performance.

Appendix A: Methodology: Executive Health and Fitness Survey

IDENTIFICATION OF COMPANIES AND EXECUTIVES

In the fall of 1986, the Exercise Physiology Laboratory staff at the UMass Medical School in Worcester, Massachusetts, conducted a national health and fitness survey of 3,111 top executives of American corporations. Their names were obtained from four sources:

1. The *Fortune* 500 list of the 500 largest U.S. industrial corporations, published in the April 28, 1986 issue of *Fortune* magazine. Companies on this annual list are ranked by total sales; more than 50% of revenues have to come from manufacturing or mining.

2. The *Inc.* 100 list of the fastest-growing publicly held companies, published in the May 1986 issue of *Inc.* magazine. Companies are ranked by the percentage increase in net sales (or total revenues) over a five-year period; sales in the base year have to be at least $100,000, but no more than $25 million.

3. The *Venture* Fast Track 100 list of the largest companies founded in the past 10 years whose founders are still in control, published in the July 1986 issue of *Venture* magazine.

4. Dun's Marketing Services lists of large and small U.S. companies in each SIC industry, categorized by number of employees. For the purposes of the research, "small" companies were defined as those with 100 to 499 employees and "large" companies as those with 500 or more employees. A random sample of 1,250 small and 1,250 large companies was selected. Based on a weighted population index, a percentage was chosen from each state to avoid possible regional bias. After duplicate listings were purged, the net list included 1,209 small companies and 1,202 large companies.

The survey questionnaire, which follows at the end of this appendix, was sent to the individual identified as the chief executive officer for each of the *Fortune, Inc.,* and *Venture* companies. The list of *Fortune* 500 CEOs was obtained from the American List Counsel. The names of *Venture* and *Inc.* CEOs came from Standard & Poor's *Register of Corporations, Directors & Executives,* Dun & Bradstreet's *Million Dollar Directory,* and telephone calls to the companies.

For the Dun's Marketing Services lists, executive titles used for mailing questionnaires were owner, partner, president, or chairman. As an additional criterion, executives had to be between the ages of 18 and 65. Dun's provided the names and addresses of the executives.

MAILINGS AND RESPONSE RATE

Three separate mailings, each a month apart, were sent to the executives. The mailings included the questionnaire, a personal letter explaining the survey and requesting participation, and a stamped, self-addressed return envelope. The first mailing brought 550 responses; the second, 330; and the third, 259, for a total of 1,139—a 37% response rate. A breakdown of the mailings and responses is as follows:

	No. Sent	No. Responses	% Response	% Total
Fortune 500 CEOs	500	128	25.6	11.2
Inc. 100 CEOs	100	46	46.0	4.0
Venture Fast Track 100 CEOs	100	27	27.0	2.4
Dun's Large-Company Executives	1,202	481	40.0	42.2
Dun's Small-Company Executives	1,209	457	37.8	40.1

DATA ANALYSIS

Information from the 1,139 completed questionnaires was entered on an IBM PC-AT computer using R-Base System V and means, standard deviations, and cross tabulations were calculated.

INTERVIEWS

Based on their responses to the questionnaire, 33 top executives from a cross section of companies and with varying fitness programs were interviewed for the project. Seven corporate fitness program administrators were interviewed separately.

SURVEY QUESTIONNAIRE

Executive Cardiofitness

COMPANY DESCRIPTORS

1. Number of employees (total employees) _____

2. Geographical location (city/state) _____

3. 1985 sales (dollars) _____

4. Type of business _____

DEMOGRAPHIC INFORMATION

5. Age (years) _____

6. Sex ☐ Male ☐ Female

7. Race
   ☐ White (Non-Hispanic)
   ☐ Black (Non-Hispanic)
   ☐ Hispanic
   ☐ Asian or Pacific Islander
   ☐ American Indian or Alaskan Native

8. Weight (lbs.) _____ 9. Height (in.) _____

10. Marital status
    ☐ Single
    ☐ Married
    ☐ Divorced/Separated
    ☐ Widowed

11. Highest level of education completed
    ☐ High school diploma or less
    ☐ Two year college
    ☐ Four year college
    ☐ M.B.A.
    ☐ Other master's degree
    ☐ Doctoral degree

12. Occupation/Title _____

13. Annual Income (annual income/income from other sources) _____ / _____

GENERAL HEALTH

14. In general, how would you rate your current health?
    ☐ Excellent
    ☐ Very Good
    ☐ Good
    ☐ Fair
    ☐ Poor

15. When did you last have a complete physical examination?
    ☐ Within the past year
    ☐ Within the last 2 years
    ☐ Within the last 3 years
    ☐ 4 or more years ago
    ☐ Never had a complete physical examination

16. During the past year, how many times have you seen or talked to a physician for medical reasons? _____

17. How many days were you sick in the past year? _____

18. Of the days you were sick during the past year, how many days did you stay home from work? _____

19. Do you know your blood pressure?
    ☐ Yes
    ☐ No
    If yes, what is it? _____
    Approximate date of last measurement (month/year) _____

20. Do you know your cholesterol level? _____
    ☐ Yes
    ☐ No
    If yes, what is it? _____
    Approximate date of last measurement (month/year) _____

21. Have you ever smoked cigarettes?
    ☐ Yes
    ☐ No
    If no, please go to question number 25.
    If yes, how many years have you smoked cigarettes? _____

22. If you are an ex-smoker, how long has it been since you smoked your last cigarette?
    _____

23. Do you currently smoke cigarettes? _____
    ☐ Yes
    ☐ No

24. If you currently smoke cigarettes, how many do you smoke per day? _____
    (cigarettes/day)

25. Please check if you have ever had any of the following conditions diagnosed by a physician, and if so, your age at the time of diagnosis.

Condition	Check if diagnosed	Age at time of diagnosis
High blood pressure........	☐	_____
Heart disease/heart attack...	☐	_____
Diabetes.................	☐	_____
Cerebrovascular disease/ stroke....................	☐	_____
Elevated cholesterol levels ...	☐	_____
Family history of heart disease in parent less than 60 years of age	☐	

26. Have you ever had an exercise stress (treadmill, bike) test?
    ☐ Yes
    ☐ No
    If yes, were any of the test results abnormal? ☐ Yes ☐ No ☐ Unsure

HEALTH ATTITUDES

27. On a scale of 1–5, how important do you consider the following factors to the maintenance of your personal health (please circle your answer).

	1 = Not important		3 = Average importance		5 = Extreme importance
Diet (less sugar, salt, fats)..........	1	2	3	4	5
Regular exercise	1	2	3	4	5
Not smoking.....................	1	2	3	4	5
Limiting alcohol consumption	1	2	3	4	5
Controlling stress.................	1	2	3	4	5
Adequate sleep	1	2	3	4	5
Allowing leisure/recreation time for self............................	1	2	3	4	5

EXERCISE

28. Do you exercise regularly?
    ☐ Yes
    ☐ No
    If no, please go to question number 34.
    If yes, how long have you participated in a regular exercise program?
    _____ years   or _____ months

29. Please check any/all of the following activities you **regularly** participate in, and the typical frequency, intensity, and duration of these activities. Please rate intensity as follows:

L = light   M = moderate   S = strenuous

Activity	Frequency (times/week)	Average duration (minutes)	Average intensity (L, M, S)
1. Racquetball			
2. Squash/handball			
3. Tennis			
singles _____			
doubles _____			
4. Stationary cycling			
5. Outdoor cycling			
6. Aerobic dance/exercise conditioning			
7. Fitness walking			
8. Jogging/running			
9. Swimming			
10. Rowing			
11. Cross-country skiing			
12. Downhill skiing			
13. Calisthenics			
14. Weight training			
free weights _____			
Nautilus type _____			
Universal _____			
15. Golf			
walk ___ cart ___			
16. Bowling			
17. Basketball			
18. Other: please specify			
_____			

30. Do you have a regular exercise time during the day?
If yes, please specify the time of day you usually exercise.
☐ Yes _____ ☐ A.M. ☐ P.M.
☐ No

31. Where do you usually exercise? (please check all that apply)
☐ In own home/outdoors
☐ In a health/racquet club
☐ In a corporate fitness exercise center
☐ At a local YMCA/recreational type setting
☐ Other: please specify _____

32. On a scale of 1–5, rate how important **each** factor is in motivating you to exercise.

	1 = unimportant		3 = average		5 = very important
Health benefits	1	2	3	4	5
Improved physical appearance	1	2	3	4	5
Improved productivity	1	2	3	4	5
Maintain/lose weight	1	2	3	4	5
Improved sense of well-being	1	2	3	4	5
Can eat more	1	2	3	4	5
Concentrate better	1	2	3	4	5
Reduce stress	1	2	3	4	5
Enjoyment of exercise	1	2	3	4	5
Better equipped to tackle personal/ professional problems	1	2	3	4	5

33. Many factors hinder a regular exercise schedule. What factors, if any, limit you from engaging in a regular exercise program? (please rate **each** factor on a scale of 1–5)

	1 = never		3 = occasionally		5 = often
Inadequate time	1	2	3	4	5
Lack of adequate facility	1	2	3	4	5
Fatigue	1	2	3	4	5
Motivation	1	2	3	4	5
Travel/disruptive schedule	1	2	3	4	5
Other:	1	2	3	4	5

Please specify _____

34. If you do not exercise, what are your reasons for not exercising? (please check all that apply)

☐ No interest in exercising
☐ Don't enjoy exercise/too boring
☐ Get enough exercise in daily work/routine
☐ Limited by health problems
☐ Adequate facilities not available
☐ Inadequate time/too busy
☐ Frequent travel
☐ Other: please specify _____

35. From where do you derive your information about health and fitness? (please check all that apply)

☐ Health/sports magazines/media
☐ Health and fitness books
☐ Exercise physiologist/fitness instructor in corporate setting
☐ Exercise instructor in health club
☐ Previous personal experience (high school coach, etc.)
☐ Personal physician
☐ Other: please specify _____

36. How does your current physical condition compare with five years ago?

☐ Better
☐ Worse
☐ Same

37. Would you like to improve your physical condition over the next five years?

☐ Yes   ☐ No

38. When did you compete in team or individual sports? (please check all that apply)

☐ High school
☐ College
☐ After college
☐ Never competed in sports

39. Do you currently compete in competitive/organized athletics?

☐ Yes
☐ No

    If yes, please specify sport: _____

DIET

40. Which of the following items do you attempt to avoid or minimize in your diet? (please check all that apply)

☐ High-cholesterol foods   ☐ Caffeine   ☐ Snacks
☐ Salt/sodium   ☐ Refined sugars/sweets   ☐ Fried foods
☐ High-fat dairy products   ☐ Red meat   ☐ Alcohol
☐ Other: please specify _____

41. How many times per week do you drink beer, wine, or hard liquor? _____ times per week

☐ Less than once per week
☐ Rarely
☐ Never

42. On these occasions, how many drinks do you usually have? A drink is 12 ounces of beer, 5 ounces of wine, or 1½ ounces of hard liquor (whiskey, gin, etc.).

☐ One
☐ Two
☐ Three
☐ Four
☐ More than four

43. How many cups of coffee or tea do you have per week? _____

44. Do you usually drink decaffeinated coffee or tea?

☐ Yes
☐ No

45. How many cans of soda do you usually drink per week? _____

46. What type of soda do you usually drink? (please check all boxes that apply)

☐ Diet/low calorie
☐ Regular
☐ Caffeinated
☐ Decaffeinated
☐ Low sodium/salt

47. Are you currently on a special diet, or have you been on a special diet at any time during the last year? (please check all that apply)

☐ No special diet   ☐ Weight loss diet   ☐ Low salt/sodium
☐ Vegetarian diet   ☐ Low cholesterol/low fat diet   ☐ Diabetes diet
☐ other: please specify _____

DIETARY INTAKE

48. Please complete the following table based on your average eating habits during the last year. For foods you eat less than once per week check "no" in the first column and do not enter anything in the other columns. For foods that you eat more than once per week, complete all columns.

Check the Foods You Eat at Least Once per Week	What Types do You Usually Eat or Drink	How Much (Approximate Portion per Meal)	Number of Times per Week
EGGS ☐ No ☐ Yes	☐ Whole egg ☐ Yolk only ☐ White only	☐ 1 egg ☐ 2 eggs ☐ 3 eggs or more	_____ times per week
MEAT ☐ No ☐ Yes (beef, pork, lamb)	☐ Lean ☐ Medium fat ☐ Fatty	☐ sm. 3 oz. ☐ med: 4–6 oz. ☐ lrg: 7 oz. or more	_____ times per week
FISH ☐ No ☐ Yes	☐ Shellfish ☐ All other types (tuna, halibut, etc.)	☐ sm: 3 oz. ☐ med: 4–6 oz. ☐ lrg: 7 oz. or more	_____ times per week
POULTRY ☐ No ☐ Yes	☐ Skin removed ☐ Skin left on	☐ sm: 3 oz. ☐ med: 4–6 oz. ☐ lrg: 7 oz. or more	_____ times per week
PRETZELS, CHIPS, NUTS ☐ No ☐ Yes	☐ Salted ☐ Unsalted	☐ sm: 1/4 cup ☐ med: 1/2 cup ☐ lrg: 1 cup	_____ times per week

DIETARY INTAKE (*continued*)

Check the Foods You Eat at Least Once per Week	What Types do You Usually Eat or Drink	How Much (Approximate Portion per Meal)	Number of Times per Week
HAM, BACON, HOT DOGS, LUNCH MEAT ☐ No ☐ Yes	☐ Processed ☐ Not processed	☐ sm: 1–2 oz. ☐ med: 3–4 oz. ☐ lrg: 5 oz. or more	_____ times per week
MILK ☐ No ☐ Yes	☐ Whole ☐ 2% ☐ 1% ☐ Skim	☐ sm: 4–6 oz. ☐ med: 6–8 oz. ☐ lrg: 9 oz. or more	_____ times per week
CHEESE ☐ No ☐ Yes	☐ Low salt/sodium ☐ Low fat ☐ Regular	☐ sm: 1–2 oz. ☐ med: 3–4 oz. ☐ lrg: 5 oz. or more	_____ times per week
BUTTER ☐ No ☐ Yes	☐ Low salt ☐ Regular	☐ sm: ½ tbs. ☐ med: 1 tbs. ☐ lrg: 1¼ tbs. or more	_____ times per week
MARGARINE ☐ No ☐ Yes	☐ Stick ☐ Tub ☐ Liquid	☐ sm: ½ tbs. ☐ med: 1 tbs. ☐ lrg: 1¼ tbs. or more	_____ times per week
VEGETABLES OR FRUIT ☐ No ☐ Yes	☐ Fresh ☐ Frozen ☐ Canned	☐ sm: ½ cup ☐ med: ¾ cup ☐ lrg: 1 cup	_____ times per week
HIGH-FIBER FOODS ☐ No ☐ Yes (rice, bran, high-fiber cereals, whole wheat breads, legumes [dried beans/peas/lentils])	Please indicate types: _____ _____ _____ _____		Amount usually eaten: ____ times/wk ____ times/wk ____ times/wk ____ times/wk

STRESS

49. How much job-related pressure do you usually experience?

☐ Very little
☐ A moderate amount
☐ Quite a bit
☐ An extreme amount

50. How much **negative** job-related stress do you usually experience?

☐ Very little
☐ A moderate amount
☐ Quite a bit
☐ An extreme amount

51. How do you feel you cope with your job-related stresses?

☐ Poorly
☐ Fairly well
☐ Moderately well
☐ Very well

52. How much **negative** stress do you experience in your personal life?

☐ Very little
☐ A moderate amount
☐ Quite a bit
☐ An extreme amount

53. How do you feel you cope with your personal stresses?

☐ Poorly
☐ Fairly well
☐ Moderately well
☐ Very well

54. Do you have any physical symptoms you relate to your stress? (if yes, please list them)

☐ Yes _____
☐ No

PROFESSIONAL LIFE

55. How many hours a week do you work? _____

56. What do you do to ensure that you reach your performance goals? (please check all that apply)

☐ Work overtime
☐ Work weekends
☐ Follow a planned program
☐ Eat properly
☐ Study and prepare
☐ Exercise
☐ Personal program for handling stress
☐ Other: (please explain) _____

57. Do you have a specific strategy (such as walking up stairs instead of using the elevator) to increase your activity level at work?

☐ Yes
☐ No   If yes, please explain _____

58. On a scale of 1–5, please rate the level of personal satisfaction you receive from **each** of the following factors (please circle your answer)

	NA = not applicable	1 = least satisfaction		3 = average satisfaction		5 = most satisfaction
Family	NA	1	2	3	4	5
Friends	NA	1	2	3	4	5
Spouse	NA	1	2	3	4	5
Children	NA	1	2	3	4	5
Religion	NA	1	2	3	4	5
Sports	NA	1	2	3	4	5
Hobbies	NA	1	2	3	4	5
Investments	NA	1	2	3	4	5
Work	NA	1	2	3	4	5
Community work	NA	1	2	3	4	5
Other, please specify ..	NA	1	2	3	4	5

59. Have you had to make any personal sacrifices to achieve success?

☐ Yes
☐ No

If yes, please explain _____

_____

_____

_____

_____

_____

Thank you very much for your time and effort in completing this questionnaire. Please feel free to comment as you wish.

Appendix B: Executive Interviews (by company)

As a follow-up to a national survey of top executives that attracted 1,139 net responses, the author interviewed 40 CEOs and senior managers representing a diverse cross section of American industry. They are listed below.

Company/Interviewee	1985 Sales ($ millions)	No. of employees	Industry
Action Products International, Inc. (Ocala, FL) Judith Kaplan, CEO	3	35	Gift/souvenir wholesaler
American Telephone & Telegraph (New York) Peter Rhinehardt, corporate vice-president Alan Colodner, director, fitness center	34,910	337,600	Communications, electronics
Appleton & Lange (Norwalk, CT) Lin Patterson, president and CEO	not available		Publishing
Ciprico, Inc. (Plymouth, MN) Ronald Thomas, chairman and former president	8	76	Manufacturing: disk controllers
Cone Communications (Boston) Carol Cone, president	1.4	55	Public relations
Adolph Coors Company (Golden, CO) William Coors, chairman Robert Rechholtz, vice-president of sales and marketing Abe Phillips, president, Coors Energy Company Max Morton, manager, wellness center	1,281	9,400	Beverages
EG&G, Inc. (Wellesley, MA) Dean Freed, vice-chairman	1,155	23,000	Manufacturing: scientific and photographic equipment

193

Company/Interviewee	1985 Sales ($ millions)	No. of employees	Industry
Federal-Mogul Corporation (Southfield, MI) T. F. Russell, chairman and CEO	895	12,453	Manufacturing: bearings, industrial/farm equipment
Fruehauf (Detroit) Robert Rowan, chairman and former CEO	2,564	26,500	Manufacturing: automotive parts and equipment
Grumman Corporation (Bethpage, NY) John Bierwirth, senior management consultant and former chairman and CEO	3,049	32,000	Aerospace
Interand Corporation (Chicago) Leonard Reiffel, Ph.D., CEO	7	92	Manufacturing: telecom- munications systems
Jacor Communications, (Cincinnati, OH) Terry Jacobs, chairman	14	300	Broadcasting
Johnson & Johnson (New Brunswick, NJ) Phillip Carnes, group chairman John Woodward, corporate secretary Frank Barker, president, Health Management, Inc. Melvin Benjamin, director, Live for Life program	6,421	74,900	Pharmaceuticals
MBI Business Centers, Inc. (Rockville, MD) Avner Parnes, former chairman and CEO	51	390	Sales: micro- computer and related products
Medical Care International, Inc. (Dallas) Donald Steen, president and CEO	35	600	Outpatient surgi- cal centers
Nashua Corporation (Nashua, NH) Charles Clough, president, chairman, and CEO	622	5,275	Manufacturing: computers and office equipment
Navistar International Corp. (Chicago)* Donald Lennox, board member and former CEO	3,752	16,836	Manufacturing: motor vehicles and parts
Norton Company (Worcester, MA) John Nelson, chairman and CEO Thomas Hourihan, vice-president of human resources	1,193	18,100	Manufacturing: abrasives and building materials
Sentry Insurance (Concord, MA) Steven Schroeder, vice-president Mike Day, vice-president, corporate communications	not available	not available	Life and casualty underwriter

Company/Interviewee	1985 Sales ($ millions)	No. of employees	Industry
Ronald Cook, corporate manager, employee wellness			
Simon & Schuster (New York)**	1,200	9,000	Publishing
Richard Snyder, chairman and CEO			
Tenneco, Inc. (Houston)	15,400	111,000	Petroleum refining
J. L. Ketelsen, chairman and CEO			
Joe B. Foster, former executive vice-president			
K. W. Reese, executive vice-president			
Kenneth L. Otto, senior vice-president			
Edward J. Bernacki, M.D., vice-president, health, environmental, medicine, and safety			
William Baun, manager, health and fitness			
Ungermann-Bass, Inc. (Santa Clara, CA)	72	100	Manufacturing: LAN systems
Ralph Ungermann, president and CEO			
Winnebago Industries (Forest City, IA)	424	2,250	Manufacturing: transportation equipment
Gerald Gilbert, former president and CEO			
Xerox Corporation (Stamford, CT)	8,948	102,396	Manufacturing: scientific and photographic equipment
Paul Allaire, president			
Craig Wright, medical director			

Source: Compiled by the author.
*Formerly International Harvester—name changed in 1986.
**1988 figures.

References

CHAPTER 1

1. The *Fortune* 500, *Fortune*. Time, Inc. April 1986.
2. The *Venture* Fast Track 100, *Venture,* May 1986.
3. The *Inc.* 100, *Inc.* Goldhirsh Group. May 1986.

CHAPTER 2

1. American Heart Association. 1983. *About your heart and exercise.* (Available from the American Heart Association.) Dallas, TX: American Heart Association.
2. American Heart Association Committee on Exercise. 1972. *Exercise training and testing of apparently healthy individuals: A handbook for physicians.* Dallas, TX: American Heart Association.
3. American Heart Association Committee on Exercise. 1975. *Exercise testing and training of individuals with heart disease or at high risk for its development: A handbook for physicians.* Dallas, TX: American Heart Association.
4. American College of Sports Medicine. 1978. *Position stand on fitness in healthy adults.* (Available through the American College of Sports Medicine.) Indianapolis, IN.
5. American College of Sports Medicine. 1986. *Guidelines for exercise testing and prescription.* 3d ed. Philadelphia: Lea & Febiger.
6. U.S. Department of Health and Human Services Public Health Service. *Facts about exercise.* (Available from USPHS.)
7. Brooks, G. A., and T. B. Fahey. 1984. *Exercise physiology: Human bioenergetics and its applications.* New York: J. Wiley & Sons.
8. Shephard, J. R. 1982. *Physiology and biochemistry of exercise.* New York: Praeger.
9. McArdle, W. D., F. I. Katch, and V. L. Katch. 1981. *Exercise physiology.* Philadelphia: Lea & Febiger.
10. Froelicher, V. F. 1983. *Exercise testing and training.* Chicago: LeJaq Publishing.
11. Cooper, K. H. 1970. *The new aerobics.* New York: Bantam.
12. Sheffeld, L. T. 1984. Exercise stress testing. In *Heart disease,* ed. Braunwald, E. Philadelphia: W. B. Saunders.
13. Astrand, P. O., and K. Rodahl. 1977. *Textbook of work physiology.* New York: McGraw-Hill, Inc.

14. President's Council on Physical Fitness. 1987. *Staying with it* (Available through the President's Council on Physical Fitness) and *Life fitness.* Irvine, CA.
15. Rippe, J. M. 1987. A winter's tale: How to prevent your exercise from becoming a statistic. *Newsweek* Health and Fitness Supplement (September).
16. Rippe, J. M. (moderator). 1987. Lifelong exercise for optimal health and fitness: Roundtable discussion. *The Physician and Sports Medicine* (October and November).
17. Kashiwa, A., and J. M. Rippe. 1987. *Fitness walking for women.* New York: G. P. Putnam and Sons.
18. Ward, A., and J. M. Rippe. 1987. *Planning your personal fitness program.* Philadelphia: J. B. Lippincott.
19. Levy, B. S., R. Goldberg, J. Rippe, and D. Love. 1984. A regular exercise program for medical students: Impact on health, personal habits and attitudes. *Journal of Medical Education* 59:596.
20. Porcari, J., R. McCarron, G. Kline, P. Freedson, A. Ward, J. Ross, and J. Rippe. 1987. Is fast walking an adequate aerobic stimulus in 30–69-year-old adults? *Physician and Sports Medicine* 15:119.
21. Ryan, A. Exercise is medicine. 1985. *Physician and Sports Medicine.* New York: McGraw-Hill, Inc.
22. Rippe, J. M., A. Ward, and P. Freedson. 1988. Walking for fitness. *Encyclopedia Brittanica* Medical and Health Annual. Chicago: Encyclopedia Brittanica, Inc.
23. Paffenbarger, R., et al. 1986. College alumni study. Physical activity, all cause mortality and longevity of college alumni. *New England Journal of Medicine* 314:605.

CHAPTER 3

1. Rippe, J. M., and W. Southmayd. 1986. *The sports performance factors.* New York: G. P. Putnam and Sons.
2. Kline, G. M., J. P. Porcari, R. Hintermeister, P. S. Freedson, A. Ward, R. F. McCarron, J. Ross, and J. M. Rippe. 1987. Prediction of VO$_2$ max from a one-mile track walk. *Medicine and Science in Sports and Exercise* 19:253.

CHAPTER 4

1. American Heart Association. 1984. *The American Heart Association cookbook.* 4th ed. New York: Ballantine Books.
2. Connor, S. J., and W. E. Connor. 1986. *The new American diet.* New York: Simon & Schuster.

3. Yetiv, J. Z. 1986. *Popular nutritional practices: A scientific appraisal.* Toledo, Ohio: Popular Medicine Press.

4. Saltman, P., J. Gurin, and I. Mothner. 1987. *The California nutrition book.* Boston: Little, Brown.

5. Brody, J. 1987. *Jane Brody's nutrition book.* 2d ed. New York: Bantam.

6. Nidetch, J. 1986. *Weight Watchers Quick Start Plus Program cookbook.* New York: New American Library.

7. The Nutrition Foundation Inc. 1984. *Present knowledge in nutrition.* 5th ed. Washington, D.C.

8. Leveille, G. A. 1985. *The Set Point diet.* New York: Ballantine.

9. Katch, F. I., and W. D. McArdle. 1977. *Nutrition, weight control and exercise.* Boston: Houghton Mifflin.

10. Clark, N. 1986. Nutrition. In *The sports performance factors,* Rippe, J. M., and W. Southmayd. New York: G. P. Putnam and Sons.

11. Rippe, J. M. 1986. A note on cholesterol. In *The Barbara Krauss Cholesterol Counter.* New York: G. P. Putnam and Sons.

12. American Cancer Society. 1979. *Proceedings of the American Cancer Society and National Cancer Institute National Conference on nutrition in cancer.* American Cancer Society reprint, 1984.

13. American Heart Association. *Heart to heart: Nutritional counseling for reduction of cardiovascular disease risk factors.* U.S. Department of Health and Human Services. NIH Publication #83-1528.

14. Gurin, J., and the editors of *American Health* magazine. 1987. Eating to excel. *American Health* (October).

15. American Heart Association. The American Heart Association diet: An eating plan for healthy Americans. (Available from the American Heart Association.)

16. American Heart Association. 1982. Rationale of the diet heart statement of the American Heart Association: Report of the nutrition committee. Circulation 65:839A.

17. American Heart Association. Eating for a healthy heart: Dietary treatment of hyperlipidemia. (Available from the American Heart Association.)

18. Grundy, S. M. 1986. Cholesterol and coronary heart disease: A new era. *JAMA* 256:2849.

19. Blank, D. W., J. M. Hoeg, M. H. Kroll, et al. 1986. The method of determination must be considered in interpreting blood cholesterol level. *JAMA* 256:2867.

20. Rifkin, B. M. 1986. Cholesterol lowering and reduction of coronary heart disease risk. *JAMA* 256:2872.

21. Grouse, L. 1986. Taking on the fat of the land: Cholesterol and health. *JAMA* 256:2873.

22. Shekelle, R. B., A. M. Shryock, O. Paul, et al. 1981. Diet, serum cholesterol, and death from coronary heart disease: The Western Electric study. *New England Journal of Medicine* 304:65.

23. Hartung, G. H., J. P. Foreyt, R. E. Mitchell, et al. 1980. Relation of diet to high density lipoprotein cholesterol in middle-aged marathon runners, joggers and inactive men. *New England Journal of Medicine* 302:357.

24. Haskell, W. L. 1984. Exercise induced changes in plasma lipids and lipoproteins. *Preventive Medicine* 13:23.

25. Lipid Research Clinics Program. 1984. The Lipid Research Clinics coronary primary prevention trial results: I. Reduction in incidence of coronary heart disease. *JAMA* 251:351.

26. Lipid Research Clinics Program. 1984. The Lipid Research Clinics coronary primary prevention trial results: II. The relationship of reduction in incidence of coronary heart disease to cholesterol lowering. *JAMA* 251:365.

27. Goldberg, L., and D. L. Elliot. 1985. The effect of physical activity on lipid and lipoprotein levels. *Medical Clinics of North America* 69:41.

28. Barness, L. A. 1986. Cholesterol and children. *JAMA* 256:2871.

29. Castelli, W. P., R. G. Garrison, T. W. F. Wilson, et al. 1986. Incidence of coronary heart disease and lipoprotein cholesterol levels: The Framingham study. *JAMA* 256:2835.

30. NIH Consensus Conference. 1984. Treatment of hypertriglyceridemia. *JAMA* 251:1196.

31. Haskell, W. L. 1984. The influence of exercise on the concentrations of triglyceride and cholesterol in human plasma. *Exercise and Sports Science Reviews* 12:205.

32. Grundy, S. M. 1986. Comparison of monounsaturated fatty acids and carbohydrates for lowering plasma cholesterol. *New England Journal of Medicine* 314:745.

33. Parton, G. H., and W. G. Squires. 1980. Exercise and HDL cholesterol in middle-aged men. *The Physician and Sports Medicine* 8:74.

34. U.S. Department of Health and Human Services, Public Health Service. Fact sheet on hyperlipoproteinemia. (Available from the information office of the National Heart, Lung, and Blood Institute.)

35. National Institutes of Health. Consensus Development Conference statement: Lowering blood cholesterol to prevent heart disease. (Available from the National Institutes of Health.)

36. Passamani, E. R. 1987. Cholesterol reduction in coronary artery bypass patients. *JAMA* 257:3271.

37. Blankenhorn, D. H., S. A. Nessim, R. A. Johnson, et al. 1987. Beneficial effects of combined cholesterol-niacin therapy on coronary atherosclerosis and coronary venous bypass grafts. *JAMA* 257:3233.

38. Superco, H. R., P. S. Bachorik, and P. D. Wood. 1986. High density lipo-protein cholesterol measurements: A help or hindrance in practical clinical medicine? *JAMA* 256:2714.

39. Levy, R. I. 1985. Lipid regulation: A new era in the prevention of coronary heart disease. *American Heart Journal* 110:1099.

40. American Cancer Society. 1984. Special report: Nutrition and cancer: Cause and prevention. Reprinted from *Ca:A Cancer Journal for Clinicians* 34:2.

41. Hughes, R. 1987. The good, the bad, and the unsaturated: Cholesterol is still public enemy no. 1. *The Walking Magazine* (July).

42. Cahill, K. 1988. Sneak attack: Fat lurks in your daily diet where you least expect it. *The Walking Magazine* (May).

43. Madar, A. 1988. Heavy facts about body fat. *The Walking Magazine* (March).

44. Surgeon general's report: U.S. Department of Health and Human Services. 1988. Nutrition for Americans. Washington, D.C.

CHAPTER 5

1. Selye, H. 1974. *Stress without distress.* New York: Signet.

2. Friedman, M., and D. Ulmer. 1984. *Treating type A behavior and your heart.* New York: Fawcett.

3. Selye, H. 1956, 1976. *The stress of life.* New York: McGraw-Hill, Inc.

4. Pelletier, K. R. 1977. *Mind as healer, mind as slayer: A holistic approach to preventing stress disorders.* New York: Delta.

5. LaGreca, G. 1985. The stress you make. *Personnel Journal* (September).

6. Hyatt, J. 1987. All stressed up and no where to go. *Inc.* (January).

7. How bosses on the brink are rescued. *Wall Street Journal,* January 28, 1981.

8. Rummel, R. M., and J. W. Rader. 1978. Coping with executive stress. *Personnel Journal* (June).

9. Many survivors of layoffs feel their turn is next: Shock, anger and illness: Like a death in the family. *Wall Street Journal,* June 19, 1982.

10. Stress, work, home relations examined in job groups study. *Wall Street Journal,* June 14, 1979.

11. Fienberg, M. R., and A. Levenstein. Stamina: The executive's ultimate resource. *Wall Street Journal,* February 22, 1982.

12. Owner's isolation can result in loneliness and high stress. *Wall Street Journal,* May 7, 1984.

13. The traveling life and the toll it takes. *New York Times,* November 29, 1981.

14. Stress increasingly seen as problem with executives more vulnerable. *Wall Street Journal,* September 28, 1982.

15. The chief executive under stress. *New York Times,* November 7, 1982.

16. DeVries, H. A. 1981. Tranquillizer effect of exercise: A critical review. *The Physician and Sports Medicine* 9:47.

17. Suters, E. T. 1986. Overdoing it. *Inc.* (November).
18. Suters, E. T. It's lonely at the top—as it should be. *Wall Street Journal,* December 30, 1985.
19. Turner, J. F. Hitting rock bottom after making it to the top. *Wall Street Journal,* August 6, 1984.
20. Benson, H., and R. L. Allen. 1980. How much stress is too much? *Harvard Business Review.* September–October.
21. Stress of American life is increasingly blamed for emotional turmoil. *Wall Street Journal,* April 2, 1979.
22. Research is indicating that stress is linked to physical illnesses. *Wall Street Journal,* April 5, 1979.
23. Perham, J. 1984. Executive health audit. *Dun's Business Month* (October).
24. McDaniel, S. W., and H. T. Heiss. Using CEO profiles in executive career planning. *Managerial Planning* (March–April).
25. Braham, J. Hazards at the top. *Industry Week,* January 21, 1985.
26. Problems of two-career families start forcing businesses to adapt. *Wall Street Journal,* July 15, 1981.
27. Condor, B. 1987. Captains of industry: Executives accustomed to running things. *Ultrasport* (January).
28. Middle-aged managers often welcome a career "plateau" a study shows. *Wall Street Journal,* March 16, 1982.
29. Job hazard: How "burn out" affects a growing number of managers. *Wall Street Journal,* April 23, 1981.
30. The marathon manager. *Management Today,* September, 1982.
31. Fienberg, M. R., and A. Levenstein. Exposing our secret passion for failure. *Wall Street Journal,* August 26, 1985.

CHAPTER 6

1. Alpert, J. S. 1985. *The heart attack handbook.* Boston: Little, Brown.
2. Chobanian, A. V. 1982. *Boston University Medical Center's heart risk book: A practical guide for preventing heart disease.* New York: Bantam.
3. Cousins, N. 1983. *The healing heart.* New York: Avon.
4. Dawber, T. R. 1980. *The Framingham study: The epidemiology of atherosclerotic disease.* Cambridge: Harvard University Press.
5. Kaplan, M. M., and J. Stamler. 1983. *Prevention of coronary heart disease: Practical management of risk factors.* Philadelphia: W. B. Saunders.
6. American Heart Association. 1983. About your heart and blood pressure. (Available from the American Heart Association.) National Center, Dallas, TX.
7. U.S. Department of Health and Human Services. 1984. National Heart,

Lung, and Blood Institute demonstration projects in workplace high blood pressure control: Summary report. NIH publication #84-2119. Washington, D.C.

8. U.S. Department of Health and Human Services. 1983. Collaboration in high blood pressure control among professionals and with the patient. (Available through the Public Health Service.) NIH.

9. U.S. Department of Health and Human Services. February 1985. The public and high blood pressure. NIH publication #85-2118. Washington, D.C.

10. U.S. Department of Health, Education and Welfare. Diagnosis and management of hypertension. DHEW publication #(NIH)79-1056.

11. American Heart Association. 1985. Coronary risk factors for the American public. (Available through the American Heart Association.) National Center, Dallas, TX.

12. American Heart Association. 1986. Heart facts. (Available from the American Heart Association.) National Center, Dallas, TX.

13. American Heart Association. 1973. *Coronary risk handbook: Estimating risk of coronary heart disease in daily practice.* (Available through the American Heart Association.) National Center, Dallas, TX.

14. American Heart Association. 1987. Fact sheet on heart attack, stroke and risk factors. (Available from the American Heart Association.) National Center, Dallas, TX.

15. U.S. Department of Health and Human Services. 1978. Fact sheet: Diabetes and cardiovascular disease. (Available from the U.S. Public Health Service.) NIH.

16. Caspersen, C. J. 1987. Protective effects of physical activity on coronary heart disease. *Morbidity and Mortality Weekly Report* 36:426.

17. Powell, K. E., P. D. Thompson, C. J. Caspersen, et al. 1987. Physical activity and the incidence of coronary heart disease. *Annual Review of Public Health* 8:253.

18. Kannel, W. B. 1984. Cardiovascular consequences of physical inactivity. *Primary Cardiology* (April).

19. Walker, W. J. 1983. Changing U.S. lifestyle and declining vascular mortality—A Retrospective. *New England Journal of Medicine* 308:649.

20. U.S. Department of Health Education and Welfare. 1978. Fact sheet: Arteriosclerosis. (Available from the U.S. Public Health Service.)

21. U.S. Department of Health and Human Services. March 1986. Report of the National Heart, Lung, and Blood Advisory Board: Heart and vascular diseases. NIH.

22. American Heart Association. 1986. Stroke facts. (Available from the American Heart Association.) National Center, Dallas, TX.

23. American Heart Association. 1984. Risk factors in stroke: A statement for

physicians by the subcommittee on risk factors and stroke of the Stroke Council. *Stroke* 15:1105.

24. American Cancer Society. 1986. Cancer facts and figures. (Available from the American Cancer Society.) New York.

25. Pollen, J. W. 1984. Lifestyle and cancer prevention: Proceedings of the fourth national conference on human values and cancer. (Available from the American Cancer Society.)

26. Gauthier, M. M. 1986. Can exercise reduce the risk of cancer? *The Physician and Sports Medicine* 14:171.

27. American Cancer Society. 1978. Proceedings of the American Cancer Society and National Cancer Institute national conference on nutrition in cancer. (Available from the American Cancer Society.) New York.

28. American Cancer Society. 1983. Proceedings of the national conference on advances in cancer therapy. (Available from the American Cancer Society.) New York.

29. Chinnici, M. Plaque control. *New York Times Magazine*, March 29, 1987.

30. American Cancer Society. 1980. Guidelines for the cancer-related check up: Recommendations and rationale. Reprinted from *Ca: A Cancer Journal for Clinicians* 30:4.

31. Douglas, B. E. 1981. Examining healthy patients: How and how often? *Mayo Clinic Proceedings* 56:57.

32. Breslow, L., and A. R. Somers. 1977. The lifetime health-monitoring program: A practical approach to preventive medicine. *New England Journal of Medicine* 296:601

33. The Canadian Task Force on Periodic Health Examination. 1979. The periodic health examination. *CMA Journal* 121:1193.

34. Frame, P. S., and S. J. Carlson. 1975. A critical review of periodic health screening using specific screening criteria. Part 1: Selected diseases of respiratory, cardiovascular, and central nervous systems. *Journal of Family Practice* 2:29.

35. Frame, P. S., and S. J. Carlson. 1975. A critical review of periodic health screening using specific screening criteria. Part 2: Selected endocrine, metabolic, and gastrointestinal diseases. *Journal of Family Practice* 2:2.

36. Frame, P. S., and S. J. Carlson. 1975. A critical review of periodic health screening using specific disease criteria. Part 3: Selected diseases of the genitourinary system. *Journal of Family Practice* 2:3.

37. Somers, A. R., F. S. Billingsly, and R. C. Safalo. Lifetime health monitoring: A whole life plan for well patient care. *Patient Care*, February 15, 1979.

38. Wechsler, H., S. Levine, R. J. Idelson, et al. 1983. The physician's role in health promotion—A survey of primary care practitioners. *New England Journal of Medicine* 308:97.

39. Okrent, D. You and the doctor: striving for a better relationship. *New York Times Magazine,* Part 2, March 29, 1987.
40. Moskal, B. S. Super clinics: Meccas for executives. *Industry Week,* September 21, 1981.
41. Johnson, H. J. 1967. Fifty years' experience with executive health examinations. *Journal of Occupational Medicine* 9 (June).
42. Fielding, J. E. 1979. Preventive medicine and the bottom line. *Journal of Occupational Medicine* 21:79.
43. Vorhani, N. O. 1985. Prevention of coronary heart disease in practice. *JAMA* 254:257.
44. Ounce of prevention is worth a pound of cure or so say proponents of the "wellness" movement. *Wall Street Journal,* September 15, 1981.
45. Rippe, J. M., and A. Ward. 1987. Initiating a fitness walking program. Philadelphia: J. B. Lippincott.
46. Freedson, P., B. Chang, J. Rippe, J. Alpert, F. Katch, and W. Kroll. Intra-arterial blood pressure measurement during graded isometric exercise. *Journal of Cardiac Rehabilitation.* (In press.)
47. Rippe, J., J. Ross, R. McCarron, J. Porcari, G. Kline, A. Ward, M. Gurry, and P. Freedson. 1986. One-mile walk time norms for healthy adults. *Medicine and Science in Sports and Exercise* 18:S21.
48. Ward, A., J. Porcari, B. Keller, P. S. Freedson, D. Hosmer, I. Ockene, J. Alpert, and J. Rippe. 1987. Estimation of VO$_2$ max from a modified Balke treadmill protocol. Presented at the American Heart Association national meeting.
49. Gettman, L. R., and M. L. Pollock. 1981. Circuit weight training: A critical review of the physiologic benefits. *The Physician and Sports Medicine* 9 (January).

CHAPTER 7

1. Ryan, A. J. (Moderator). 1980. Employee fitness programs: A roundtable discussion. *The Physician and Sports Medicine* 5:63.
2. Bjurstrom, L. A., and N. G. Alexiou. 1978. A program of heart disease intervention for public employees: A five year report. *Journal of Occupational Medicine* 20:521.
3. U.S. Department of Health and Human Services. 1981. Cardiovascular primer for the workplace. NIH publication #81-2210 (January).
4. President's Council on Physical Fitness and Sports. 1980. Health and fitness: The corporate view. Special report on employee fitness in 1980. (Available through the President's Council on Physical Fitness.) Washington, D.C.
5. Wheater, K. 1986. Corporate fitness: Businesses are finding out that employee fitness is a great investment. *Fitness Now* (Summer).

6. Bernacci, E. J., and W. B. Baun. 1984. The relationship of job performance to exercise adherence in a corporate fitness program. *Journal of Occupational Medicine* 26:529.

7. Behrens, R. A. Wellness in Small Business (Washington Business Group on Health, Wellness Series). (Available through W.B.G.H.) Washington, D.C.

8. Corporate America is on the move—in track shorts. *Christian Science Monitor*, November 30, 1982.

9. Fifteen of the nation's finest: From L. L. Bean to General Dynamics the word in the working world is wellness. *Ultrasport*, January 1987.

10. Pumping iron in executive suites: The health and fitness industry jogs into the workplace. *Venture*, January 1985.

11. Workstyle *Inc.*, January 1986.

12. Fitness fever: Everybody into the company gym. *Dun's Review*, November 1980.

13. Executive fitness aids corporate health. *International Management*, February 1980.

14. Shaping up the corporate image. *New York Times*, October 7, 1979.

15. A fitness center for professionals. *New York Times*, January 3, 1985.

16. Fit employees fatten the bottom line. *Inc.*, February 1982.

17. Shephard, R. J., M. Cox, and P. Corey. 1981. Fitness program participation: Its affect on worker performance. *Journal of Occupational Medicine* 23:359.

18. Kobasa, S. C., and R. J. Hilker. 1982. Executive work perceptions and the quality of working life. *Journal of Occupational Medicine* 24:25.

19. Washington Business Group on Health. Employment based health promotion: A wise investment: A private sector review. Presented to the subcommittee on compensation and employee benefits. U.S. House of Representatives, April 15, 1986. (Available through the W.B.G.H.) Washington, D.C.

20. Rosen, R., and C. Freedman. 1987. Developing healthy companies through human resources management. Prepared for the Washington Business Group on Health as part of Worksite Wellness Series. (Available through the W.B.G.H.) Washington, D.C.

21. Blue Cross/Blue Shield. Building a healthier company. (Available through Blue Cross/Blue Shield, the President's Council on Physical Fitness and Sports, and the American Association of Fitness Directors in Business and Industry.) Chicago: Blue Cross Association.

22. Rosen, R. H. 1985. What really ails employees? *Training and Development Journal* (December).

23. Baun, W. B., E. J. Bernacci, and S. P. Tsai. 1986. A preliminary investigation: Effect of a corporate fitness program on absenteeism and health care costs. *Journal of Occupational Medicine* 28:18.

24. Herzlinger, R. E., and J. Schwartz. How companies tackle health care costs:

Parts 1, 2, and 3. *Harvard Business Review* July–August 1985; September–October 1985; January–February 1986.

25. Shephard, R. J., P. Corey, P. Renzland, et al. 1982. The influence of an employee fitness and lifestyle modification program upon health care costs. *Canadian Journal of Public Health* 73:259.

26. When a major illness befalls key employee entire firm can suffer. *Wall Street Journal,* October 6, 1983.

27. Companies fight back against soaring costs of medical coverage. *Wall Street Journal,* May 10, 1978.

28. Weis, W. L. 1984. No smoking. *Personnel Journal* (September).

29. Walsh, D. C. 1984. Corporate smoking policies: A review and analysis. *Journal of Occupational Medicine* 26:17.

30. Kent, D. C., and L. Cenci. 1982. Smoking and the workplace: Tobacco smoke health hazards to the involuntary smoker. *Journal of Occupational Medicine* 24:469.

31. The drive to kick smoking at work. *Fortune,* September 15, 1986.

32. Fielding, J. E. 1985. Smoking: Health effects and control. Parts 1 and 2. *New England Journal of Medicine* 313:491, 555.

33. American Heart Association. 1986. Public policy on smoking and health: Toward a smoke free generation by the year 2000. (Available from the American Heart Association.) Reprinted in *Circulation* 73:381A.

34. Nicotine: Harder to kick than heroin. *New York Times Magazine,* March 29, 1987.

35. Rosenthal, A. M. Terrific bonus for smokers. *New York Times,* April 26, 1987.

36. Donoghue, S. 1977. The correlation between physical fitness, absenteeism and work performance. *Canadian Journal of Public Health* 68:201.

37. Seamonds, B. C. 1982. Stress factors and their effect on absenteeism in a corporate employee group. *Journal of Occupational Medicine* 24:393.

38. Pelletier, K. R. 1984. *Healthy people in unhealthy places: Stress and fitness in work.* Lawrence, N.Y.: Merloid.

39. Cunningham, R. M. 1982. Wellness at work: A report on health and fitness programs for employees of business and industry. (An Inquiry Book for Blue Cross/Blue Shield).

40. Parkinson, R. S., et al. 1982. *Managing health promotion in the workplace: Guidelines for implementation and evaluation.* Palo Alto, CA: Mayfield.

41. YMCA of the USA. 1987. Health enhancement for America's workforce. (Available through the Program Store YMCA of the USA.)

CHAPTER 8

1. Kleinfield, N. R. What it takes: The life of a CEO. *New York Times Magazine,* December 1, 1985.

2. Lessons from late bloomers. *Fortune,* August 31, 1987.

3. Many executives complain of stress, but few want less pressured jobs. *Wall Street Journal,* September 29, 1982.

4. Profile of typical CEO shows great job satisfaction. *Industry Week,* May 28, 1984.

5. Weighty job of chief executive. *New York Times,* September 8, 1982.

6. Love of work, not money, motivates top executives, a survey finds. *Wall Street Journal,* May 6, 1986.

7. Wills, K. J. An explorer charts passages of the executive mind. *New York Times,* March 6, 1983.

8. Galbraith, J. K. Corporate man. *New York Times,* January 26, 1984.

9. The bottom line: Despite the dangers, more executives are using cocaine at work and play. *Wall Street Journal,* April 21, 1986.

10. Why are some managers top performers? A researcher picks out 16 characteristics. *Wall Street Journal,* January 21, 1983.

11. The workaholic boss: An 18 hour day menace. *Wall Street Journal,* May 10, 1982.

12. Eiton, M. T. 1969. The mental health of the older executive. *Geriatrics* (May).

13. Goleman, D. Irrational executives: Analysts offer a new view. *New York Times,* May 1, 1984.

14. Goleman, D. Successful executives rely on own kind of intelligence. I.Q. can't explain achievement but thinking style can. *New York Times,* July 31, 1984.

15. Hey boss, did you see this story about—oops, nothing boss. *Wall Street Journal,* July 12, 1985.

16. Executives more self-confident, study finds. *Los Angeles Times,* October 25, 1983.

Index

Absenteeism
  and corporate fitness programs,
    144, 153
  smoking, 148
Acceptance, and stress management,
  114
Activities, survey results, 3–4, 15
Addiction
  caffeine, 88
  smoking, 124
  see also Alcohol; Smoking;
    Substance abuse programs;
    Tobacco Dependence Disorder
Adrenaline, 101
Advisors, 167–168
Aerobics by K. Cooper, 32
Age 30–39
  body fat, 135–136
  counseling, 139
  fitness assessment, cardiovascular,
    134
  fitness prescription, 137
  health evaluation, 132
  immunization status, 132
  laboratory tests, 133–134
  musculoskeletal examination, 136
  self-examination, 137
  vision screening, 132
Age 40–49
  body fat, 136
  counseling, 139
  fitness assessment, cardiovascular,
    134–135
  fitness prescription, 138
  health evaluation, 132–133
  laboratory tests, 134

  musculoskeletal examination, 136
  self-examination, 137
  vision screening, 132
Age 50 and older
  body fat, 136
  counseling, 139–141
  fitness assessment, cardiovascular,
    135
  fitness prescription, 138
  glaucoma testing, 132
  health evaluation, 133
  immunizations, 132
  laboratory tests, 134
  musculoskeletal examination, 136
  self-examination, 137
AIDS counseling, 130
Alcohol, 88–90
  calories in, 89
  cancer, 94
  health benefits, 88–89
  laboratory tests, 133
  risks, 88
  stroke, 25
  survey results, 2, 89–90
  vitamin absorption, 90
Alertness, training effect, 20
Allergy, passive smoking, 124
American Cancer Society
  exercise and cancer, 127
  health evaluation, 129
  nutrition and cancer, 93
American College of Sports
  Medicine, 19, 36
American Heart Association
  aerobic exercise, 19, 26
  cholesterol guidelines, 75, 77

American Heart Association
 (*continued*)
 cholesterol screening, 150
 fat guidelines, 82
 hypertension screening, 151
 salt guidelines, 84
 starting exercise, 36
American Sports Data, Inc., 49
Angina
 defined, 22
 and heart disease, 21
 passive smoking, 124
Anthony, S. B., 172
Anxiety, and exercise, 112
Appearance
 diet, 74
 strength training, 61–62
 weight control, 91
Arm, injury, 61
Arrhythmia, 102, 103
Arterial disease
 and diabetes, 127
 see also Heart disease
Arteriosclerosis, 21, 22
Arthritis, 105–106, 136
Arthur D. Little, 144
Aspartame. *See* Nutrasweet™
Association for Fitness in Business,
 152
Atherosclerosis, 76
Athletics
 nutrition, 94–96
 success, 170–171
 survey results, 94

Back pain. *See* Injuries, back
Back, stretching, 67
Balance, and stress management,
 115, 116
Basal metabolic rate (BMR), 92
Bernacki, E. J., 140
Blood chemistry, 133

Blood, occult, 133
Blood pressure
 survey results, 1
 walking, 112
 warm-up/cool-down, 66
 see also Hypertension
Blood sugar, 86, 96, 133
Boredom, 56, 170
Bowel problems, fiber intake, 83
Breakfast, 96
Breathing, control of, 100
Brody, J., 83
Bruce Protocol, 45
Bruce, R., 45
Budgets, and stress levels, 107
BUN. *See* Kidney function testing
Burkitt, D., 82
Business meals, and maintaining diet
 balance, 71
Business pressure, and exercise, 14
Business size, survey results, 153
Butter, as cholesterol source, 76

Caffeine, 88
Caliper, skinfold, 135, 136
Calories
 alcohol, 89
 fiber, 83
 obesity, 92
 snacking, 71–72
Calves, stretching, 67
Canadian Air Force Exercises, 32
Canadian Life Assurance Co., 144
Cancer
 alcohol, 88
 attitudes toward, 126
 caffeine, 88
 diet, 126
 early detection, 133
 exercise, 126
 inactivity, 126

life-style, 126
mortality, 125
nutrition, 93–94
nutritional therapy, 94
risk, 139
self-examination, 126
smoking, 16, 88, 124, 126
stress, 105
Cancer, breast, 137
Cancer, colon, 81, 82–83
Cancer, rectal, 82
Cancer, skin, 137
Cancer, testicular, 137
Cannon, W., 100
Capacity, aerobic, 39–45
Carbohydrate loading, 95
Carbohydrates, and athletic training, 95
Cardiac arrest, 102–103
    see also Heart attack; Heart disease
Cardiovascular fitness, assessment, 134–135
Cardiovascular system, cooling down, 18
Center for Health and Fitness, University of Massachusetts Medical School, 129
Centers for Disease Control, 22
CHD (coronary heart disease). *See* Heart disease
Cheese, as cholesterol source, 76
Chest pain
    diagnosing, 104
    and stress, 103–104
Children
    scheduling time for, 120
    and women executives, 168–169
    see also Family
Chocolate, 81, 88
Cholesterol
    caffeine, 88
    defined, 76

diet reform, 72–73
exercise tolerance testing, 134
function, 76
"good" vs. "bad," 77
guidelines, 75
heart disease, 16, 22–23, 77, 127
obesity, 91
physicians' attitudes, 75
saturated fats, 81
screening, as corporate benefit, 150
snacking, 71–72
sources, 75–76, 78–79
stroke, 25
subfractions, 77
testing, 133, 134
vitamins, 91
Cholesterol level
    assessing, 77
    lowering, 80
Chores, outdoor, 6
Cleveland Clinic, 129
Coconut oil, 81
Colds, and vitamin C, 90
College Alumni Study, 16, 26, 50
Commandments, Corporate, 161–162
Communication, and fitness centers, 145
Community concerns, 173
Companies, small, managing, 166–167
Company type, and stress levels in senior executives, 106
Competition, and stress levels, 108
Concentration, and stress management, 113
Constipation, 82
Control, sense of, 20
Cool-down periods, 18, 38, 66
Cooper, K., 32
Coronary artery disease, and cholesterol subfractions, 77

Corporate culture, 145–146
Counseling
  in corporate fitness program, 152
  health evaluation, 131, 139–140
  life-style, 130
Coworkers, sedentary, 10–11
Cramps, preventing, 96
Creatinine. *See* Kidney function
  testing
Cycling, 55–58

Dairy products, and fats, 82
Data analysis, 181
Death of parent, and regular
  exercise, 10
Dehydration, 95
Delegation, and stress management,
  115
Deltoids, stretching, 67
Dental health, 131
  see also Tooth decay
Depression, and stress, 104–105
Diabetes, 80, 127–128
Diet
  books, 91
  cancer, 93–94, 126
  cholesterol, 75–80
  control strategies, 73–74
  diabetes, 128
  hypertension, 24
  knowledge as power, 75
  out-of-date information, 33, 74–75
  reasons to control, 74
  survey results, 1, 2, 70
  travel, 70–71, 73
Diet guidelines
  alcohol, 88
  caffeine, 88
  carbohydrates, 95
  cholesterol, 77–80
  fats, 80–82

fiber, 82–83
salt, 83–85
sugar, 85
vitamins, 90–91
Dieting, yo-yo, 92–93
Digestion, control of, 100
Dinner, 96
Diphtheria, 132
Discipline, perception of, and
  alcohol, 90
Discrimination, 170–172
Diverticulosis, 82, 83
Divorce, and stress, 118
Dizziness, 25
Dodson, J., 101
Drinks, athletic "performance," 95
"Drop-off" effect after regular
  exercise, 13

Egg yolk, as cholesterol source, 76
Electrocardiogram, 134
Elimination, and fiber, 82
Emotions, 169
Endurance, 20, 53, 61, 138
  assessing, 63
  carbohydrate loading, 95
  defined, 62
Energy, and diet, 74, 86, 94–95
Energy production, aerobic, 17–18
Energy production, anaerobic, 17–
  18
Entrepreneurs
  and boredom, 170
  stepping aside, 166–167
  and stress levels, 106–107
Ethics, 174
ETT (exercise tolerance test), 34–36,
  134
Executives
  desk-chair, 1, 2–3
  women, 168–173

Exercise
aging, 175–176
cancer, 126
classes, 151
college-to-job transition, 130
consistency vs. intensity, 50
corporate fitness programs, 151–152
frequency, survey results, 4
increasing, 177
information, out-of-date, 30, 33, 36
information, sources, 30–31
logistics and ease, 4
mental benefits, 112
performance, 177–178
perspective, 115
planning, 178
prescription, 134
psychological value, 46
starting, 37–38
age 50 and older, 138
stress management, 112–113
Exercise, aerobic
activities, 18–19
beginning or increasing, 19
blood cholesterol levels, 77
calories consumed, 93
cholesterol, 80
cornerstone of program, 38–60
defined, 17–18, 38–39
most common, 18–19
prescription for, 137–138
strength training, 61
survey results, 93
training effect, 19–20
warm-up/cool-down, 18
weight control, 92–93
see also Energy production, aerobic
Exercise, anaerobic, 18
Exercise, musculoskeletal,
prescription for, 137–138

Exercise Physiology Laboratory,
University of Massachusetts
Medical School, 138
Exercise program
projected growth, 49
seven steps, 33–69
structuring, 27–28, 32–33 (see also
Exercise, regular)
Exercise, regular
executives' commitment to, 2
lapses from, 7–8
misconceptions about, 26–27
motivation, 8–11, 14, 26
obstructions to, 13–16, 28–29
risk of vascular disease, 25–26
stopping, 13
and success, 2
survey results, 1, 2, 14
timing, 12–13
travel, 11
see also Exercise program

Family
and business pressures, 118–119,
168–169
compensating for demands on,
120–121
scheduling time for, 119, 120
supportive, 117–118
Fat
cancer, 94
fiber, 83
health risks, 80–81
sources, 81
sugar, 86
types, 81
Fat, body
assessment, 135–136
losing and regaining, 92–93
Fat, monounsaturated, 81
Fat, saturated, 76, 81

Fat, unsaturated, 81
Fatigue, and stress, 104
Feminist movement, 172
Fiber
    bars, 91
    cancer, 94
    defined, 82
    insoluble, 82–83
    soluble, 82, 83
    sources, 83, 84
    survey results, 82
    types, 82
Finances, and stress levels, 106–107
Fish, as cholesterol source, 76
Fish oil pills, 91
FIT (frequency, intensity, and time),
    19
Fitness, cardiovascular
    and jogging, 46
    and rowing, 58
    and walking, 49–50
    see also Capacity, aerobic
Fitness level, identifying, 38
Fitness prescription, 137–138
Fitness program
    and strength training, 60–61
    see also Exercise program
Fitness program, average
    cycling, 57
    jogging, 47
    rowing, 59
    swimming, 54
    walking, 51
    weight training, 65
Fitness program, corporate, 142–
    144, 143–147, 153
    management support, 155
    small firms, 152–153
Fitness program, expert
    cycling, 57, 58
    jogging, 48
    rowing, 60

    swimming, 54
    walking, 52
    weight training, 65
Fitness program, maintenance
    jogging, 48
    rowing, 60
    swimming, 55
    walking, 52
Fitness program, starter
    cycling, 56
    jogging, 47
    rowing, 59
    swimming, 53
    walking, 51
    weight training, 65
Fitness walking, 49–52
Fixx, J., 34
Flexibility. See Stretching
Flexibility testing, 68–69
Flu shots, 132
Focus, mental, 66
Foods
    cholesterol content, 78–79
    eating systems, 91
    processed, and fats, 82
    processed, and salt intake, 85
    see also Calories; Dairy products;
        Diet; Diet guidelines; Dieting;
        Fats; Fiber; Fish; Meats; Salt;
        Shellfish; Snacks
Foster equations, 45
Friedman, M., 102
Friends, 121

Gallup (market research), 49
Gastrointestinal disease, and
    vitamins, 90
Glaucoma, 132
    see also Tonometry
Glycogen, 95
Goals, setting, 2, 5–6
Groin, stretching, 67

Harvard Step Test, 39
HDL (high-density lipoprotein), 77, 80
Headache, and stress, 104
Health
  contributing factors, survey results, 2
  current, survey results, 1
Health care costs, 143
Health clubs, and corporate fitness programs, 151, 154
Health evaluation
  age 0–30, 130
  age 30–39, 132
  age 40–49, 132–133
  age 50 and older, 133
  communication with physician, 129
  as corporate benefit, 147–148
  defined, 129
  frequency and timing, 128–129, 130–131
  guidelines, 129, 131, 132–133
  see also Physical exams
Health and fitness, as corporate issue, 143
Health, and life-style, 122–123
Hearing tests, 133
Heart attack, 125
  see also Cardiac arrest; Heart disease
Heart catheterization, 35
Heart conditioning, 19–20
Heart disease, 9–10, 16–17
  aerobic exercise, 20
  age of onset, 21
  alcohol, 89
  atherosclerosis, 76
  caffeine, 88
  cholesterol, 75, 77, 80, 127
  diabetes, 127
  early detection, 133

ETT as screening test, 35
  exercise tolerance testing, 135
  family history, 127
  fats, 80
  hypertension, 127
  morbidity and mortality, 21
  muscle efficiency, 20
  prevalence of, 21
  regular exercise, 25–26, 50
  risk factors, 22–24, 127, 139
  risk reduction programs, as corporate benefit, 148–151
  smoking, 124, 127
  stress, 102–104
Heart, life expectancy of, 19–20
Heart rate
  checking, 37
  maximum, 36–37
  stress, 102
  warm-up/cool-down, 66
  see also Training, target zone
Heart rate, resting
  control of, 100
  determining, 36
  recommended, 19–20
  training effect, 26
Hematocrit, 133–134
Hemorrhoids, 82, 83
Hiring
  obesity, 74
  personal lives, 117
Home, as refuge from business pressure, 117–118
Honor Thy Boss, 162
"How Companies Tackle Health Care Costs" (Harvard Business Review, 1985), 143
Hypertension
  cause, 24
  defined, 23–24
  diet reform, 72–73
  exercise tolerance testing, 134

Hypertension (*continued*)
  heart disease, 16, 127
  as heart disease risk factor, 22–24
  obesity, 91
  other risk factors, 24
  regular exercise, 25–26
  salt, 85
  screening, as corporate benefit,
    150–151
  stroke, 25

Image
  alcohol, 90
  smoking, 125
Immune system, and stress, 106
Immunization, 132
Inactivity
  avoiding, 175
  cancer, 126
  heart disease, 22–23
  obesity, 92
  stroke, 25
Injuries
  assessment, 130, 136
  cycling, 55
  fitness prescription, 138
  prevention, 136, 152
  stretching, 64, 69
  swimming, 53
  walking, 50
  weight training, 61
Injuries, arm, 61
Injuries, back, 9, 58, 61
Injuries, leg, 61
Injuries, orthopedic, 49
Insomnia, and stress, 104
Interviews, 182
Ischemia, 35
  see also TIA

Job, knowing, 161–162
Job performance, 17

Jogging, 45–49
  and back pain, 61
  and travel, 5, 46
Joint
  flexibility, measuring, 69
  inflammation, and stress, 105–106
  injury, 53, 55, 136 (*see also*
    Injuries)

Kidney function testing, 133
Kipling, R., 164
Know Thy Job, 161–162
Know Thyself, 163

Laboratory tests, 133–134
Layoffs, and stress, 109
LDL (low-density lipoprotein), 77, 81
Leadership, and success, 166
Leg
  injuries, 61
  stretching, 67
Leisure/recreation, survey results, 2
Leverage, and success, 162
Life expectancy
  alcohol, 89
  at age 65, 141
  exercise, 16, 26
  of heart, 19–20
  smoking, 124
  weight control, 91
Life-style
  and cancer, 126
  counseling, 130
  and health, 122–123
Lipoprotein, 77
Liver function testing, 133
Loneliness, and depression, 105
Longfellow, H. W., 157
Looking back, and stress, 114
Loomis, W., 143

Loyalty, 166, 169–170
Luck, and success, 160–161
Lunch, 89, 96

Mammography, 133, 134
Management skills, 163–167
Marathons, and carbohydrate
    loading, 95
Mayo Clinic, 129
Meat
    fats, 81
    red, as cholesterol source, 75–76
    see also Fish; Shellfish
Medical education, and exercise
    information, 31
Mental health, and stress, 104–105,
    112
Mentors, 167–168
Menus, executive dining rooms, 73
Methodology, 180–182
Milk, as cholesterol source, 76
Minerals, 90–91
Money, as motivation, 175
Mood, and exercise, 112
Morale, and corporate fitness
    programs, 144–145, 153
Mortality
    cancer, 125
    life-style, 123
    smoking, 124
Muscle
    efficiency, 20
    groups, defined, 61
    loss in dieting, 92
Musculoskeletal examination, 136

National Cholesterol Education Program
    Expert Panel Report, 75
National Institute of Mental Health,
    124

National Institutes of Health, 26, 75,
    77
National Sporting Goods
    Association, 49
Neck, stretching, 66
Negotiations, and stress, 110
Nervous system
    autonomic, 100
    parasympathetic, 100
    sympathetic, 100–101
    voluntary, 100
Nicotine addiction, 124
Nutrasweet™ (aspartame), 87
Nutrition
    out-of-date information, 94
    see also Diet
"Nutrition and Cancer: Causes and
    Prevention," 93–94

Obesity
    cancer, 94
    fats, 81
    heart disease, 22–23
    hypertension, 24
    prejudice against overweight
        executives, 74
    stroke, 25
    sugar, 86
    see also Weight control
Opinions, soliciting, 164, 165
Organization, 158

Paffenbarger, R. S., Jr., 16, 26
Palm oil, 81
Palpitations, and stress, 102
Parties, business-related, 90, 158–159
People, managing, 163–166,
    169–170
Performance
    athletic, 94–96

Performance (*continued*)
  diet, 74, 94–96
  exercise, 177–178
  personal lives, 117
  strategies, survey results, 157
  stress, 101
Periodontal disease, 86
Perseverance, 157–159, 172–173
Personal lives
  and hiring, 117
  shielding, 117
Personnel
  fitness, 143, 144
  morale, 144–145, 153
  stress, 108–109, 110
Perspective. *See* Balance
Peter Principle, 101
Physical exams
  need for, 34–36
  survey results, 1
  see also Health evaluation
Physician, communication with, 129, 139, 141
Physicians, and exercise information, 30–32
Physiology of exercise, 17–18
Planning
  for exercise, 178
  for the future, 175
  and stress management, 114–115
Plant closing, and stress, 109
Pneumovax vaccine, 132
Poultry, as cholesterol source, 76
Power, defined, 62
Priorities, setting, 158, 159
Pritikin diet and exercise plan, 72
Pritikin, N., 72
Promotion
  obesity, 74
  stress, 109–110
Protein, in athletic training, 94–95

Pulse. *See* Heart rate
Push-ups, 63

Quadriceps, stretching, 67

Reagan, R., 85
Recruitment, and fitness programs, 144, 146
Rectal cancer, 82
Rectal examination, 133
Respect, maintaining, 165–166
Respiratory infection, and passive smoking, 124
Responsibility, and stress levels, 108
Rest, and perspective, 115
Retirement, 175
Risk factors
  alcohol, 88
  cancer, 139
  genetic, 127–128
  heart disease, 22–24, 127, 139
  hypertension, 24
  stroke, 25
Risk taking, and success, 161
Rockport Fitness Walking Test©, 39, 50
Rosenman, R. H., 102
Rowing, 7, 58–60
Running. *See* Jogging

Saccharine, 87
Salt
  as acquired taste, 84
  average consumption, 83–84
  and hypertension, 85
  shakers, 85
  survey results, 85
  tablets, 94, 96
Satisfaction, survey results, 117, 176
Scandals, "insider trading," 174

Scheduling family time, 119, 120
Self-discipline, and smoking, 125
Self-examination, 126, 137
Self image
  and exercise, 11
  and strength training, 61–62
  and stress management, 114
Self-knowledge, 163
Self, managing, 163
Self-reliance, and stress
    management, 114
Selye, H., 100
"Set point," and weight control, 92
Shellfish, as cholesterol source, 76
Shoulder, stretching, 67
Showers, and corporate fitness
    programs, 151
Sick days, survey results, 1–2
Side, stretching, 67
Sigmoidoscopy, 133
Sit-ups, 63
Sleep, survey results, 2
Smoking, 16, 123–125
  absenteeism, 148
  addiction, 124
  alcohol, 88
  cancer, 124, 126
  exercise tolerance testing, 134
  heart disease, 22–23, 124, 125,
    127
  life expectancy, 124
  mortality, 124
  passive, 124, 148
  stopping, 124–125
  stroke, 25
  survey results, 1, 2, 123
  Tobacco Dependence Disorder,
    124
  workplace, 123, 148–149
Smoking cessation programs, as
    corporate benefit, 148–150
Snacks, 71

salt intake, 85
  sugar, 85
Social responsibility, 173
Sodium intake, 24
  see also Diet; Salt
Soft drinks
  athletic "performance," 95
  caffeine, 88
  sugar intake, 86–87
  see also Alcohol
Speech, loss of, 25
Stamina, and training effect, 20
Stepping aside, 166–167, 175
Stereotypes, breakdown of, 170–172
Stomach pain, and stress, 104
Strength
  abdominal, back and leg, 58
  checking, 63
  defined, 62
  upper body, 53
Strength training
  frequency, 64
  necessity for, 60–61
  out-of-date information, 62
  rate of gain, 64
  sequencing, 61, 64–65
  and stretching, 66
Stress, 22
  balancing business and family
    demands, 118–119
  defined, 100
  and the heart, 102–104
  and hypertension, 24
  literature on, 98
  manifestations, 100–102
  and medical problems, 101–106
  reduction, 8–9, 99, 111–112, 152
  senior executives, 98–99
  survey results, 2, 98–99
  testing, 34–36 (see also ETT)
Stress, business
  management strategies, 111–116

Stress, business (*continued*)
  mental health, 104–105
  personal factors as counterbalance,
    117
  self-inflicted, 110–111
  sources, 106–111
  by type of firm, 106
Stress, personal
  divorce, 118
  management strategies, 116–121
  survey results, 116–117
Stretching
  developing a program, 69
  exercises, 66–67
  flexibility, 38, 64–66
  testing, 68–69
  see also Cool-down periods; Warm-
    up periods
Stroke, 23, 25, 127
Substance abuse programs, in
    corporate fitness programs,
    152
Success
  athletic, 170–171
  and leadership, 166
  and leverage, 162
  and luck, 160–161
  and regular exercise, 2
  and risk taking, 161
  and talent, 159–160
  and timing, 162
Sugar
  energy level, 94, 96
  obesity, 86
  in "performance" drinks in
    training, 95
  sources, 85, 87
  survey results, 86
Survey
  mailings and responses, 181
  participants, identifying, 180–
    181

questionnaire, 183–192
Survey results
  activities, 15
  ages, 107–108
  alcohol, 2
  athletics, 94
  blood pressure, 1
  business stress, 111
  caffeine, 88
  cholesterol levels, 74, 76
  company size, 153
  current health, 1
  cycling, 55
  dental health, 131
  diabetes, 128
  diet, 1, 2, 70
  executive stress, 98–99
  exercise frequency, 4
  fiber, 82
  health attitudes, 14
  health factors, 2
  jogging, 45–46
  leisure/recreation, 2
  marital status, 117–118
  motivation factors, 14
  performance strategies, 157
  physical exams, 1
  regular exercise, 1, 2, 14
  rowing, 58
  salt, 85
  satisfaction, 117
  sick days, 1–2
  sleep, 2
  smoking, 1, 2, 123
  strength training, 62
  stress
    business, 106
    manifestations, 104
    personal, 116–117
  sugar, 86
  swimming, 52–53
  walking, 49